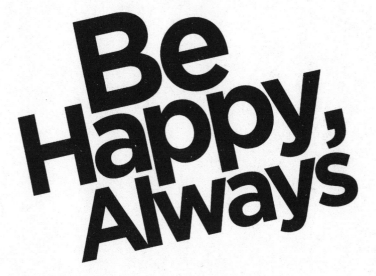

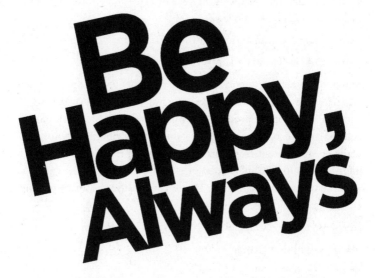

Be Happy, Always

Simple Practices for Overcoming Life's Challenges and Living Each Day with Joy

XANDRIA OOI

Mango Publishing

CORAL GABLES

Cover Design: Cheah Wei Chun from Clanhouse

Layout Design: Jermaine Lau

For permission requests, please contact the publisher at:

Mango Publishing Group
2850 S Douglas Road, 2nd Floor
Coral Gables, FL 33134 USA
info@mango.bz

For special orders, quantity sales, course adoptions and corporate sales, please email the publisher at sales@mango.bz. For trade and wholesale sales, please contact Ingram Publisher Services at customer.service@ingramcontent.com or +1.800.509.4887.

Be Happy, Always: Simple Practices for Overcoming Life's Challenges and Living Each Day with Joy

Library of Congress Cataloging
ISBN: (p) 978-1-64250-039-4 (e) 978-1-64250-040-0
LCCN: 2019944140

BISAC category code: SEL016000—SELF-HELP / Personal Growth / Happiness

Printed in the United States of America

To my mother, who is my most treasured gift and absolute blessing in life.

Content by Chapter

Content by Title

CHAPTER 3 - COMMUNICATING POSITIVELY WITH DIFFICULT PEOPLE

CHAPTER 5: LIVING WITH JOY, POSITIVITY AND GRATITUDE

Content by Subject

Introduction

When I first started writing this book, my intention was to write
about happiness. However, the more time I spent on developing
the chapters and titles, the more I realized that perhaps the book
is about *unhappiness,* for it is when we know how to navigate
through the unhappy moments in life that we can truly be
happy. This is why all five chapters in this book delve deep into
heartache, pain, hurt, depression, communication problems, and
relationship difficulties. These are all challenges that *every single
one of us* is likely to experience at one time or another, and it's
hard to not feel frustrated and upset when life isn't going the way
we hope it will.

The objective of this book is to help you build the skills
and strength to work through the challenging, difficult, and
uncomfortable times in life, because it is only then that you can
find peace.

Even when we have a great career and a wonderful relationship,
we might feel like something is missing or that our life isn't
fulfilled. Sometimes, we can start off incredibly happy with our
lives, and then after some time goes by, the problems that creep
in make our life feel incredibly exhausting. We all understand
that perfection doesn't exist, yet often we can't help but despair
when life is far from perfect. This is why it's so important for us
to understand how to take responsibility for our happiness even
in the toughest of times, because we don't want our happiness
to always be at the mercy of "what happens to us." This is why
many cannot find fulfilment—we will only learn how to be fulfilled
through the ups and downs of life.

Throughout the different chapters of this book, you'll find that
I define happiness as much more than just a feeling. You'll read
stories of how it is possible to still be happy even when life throws
us a curveball because there are practices that we can embrace
to build an incredibly solid foundation to help us weather the
storms. It is when we understand how to not suffer and how to
be at peace that we can cultivate the loving relationships we want,

as well as genuinely enjoying going to work and interacting with people without negativity, stress, or anxiety.

I've written this book so that it can be experienced in four different ways, and I highly recommend that you read its sections in this order for the most rewarding experience:

1. For your first read, experience the book in sequence from beginning to end, so that it provides a holistic understanding of how to overcome challenges in life to be happy.

2. Each section is also a self-contained lesson, so after your first read, you can flip to the individual piece that you feel compelled to read again.

3. Every title also serves as a quote. Once you've read the entire book, you can flip to the quotes that serve as a quick reminder of the philosophies you'd like to embrace in life.

4. There are three tables of content in this book. This first arranged by chapter, the second by title and the third by subject. This is so that if you'd like to actively practice happiness after you've finished the book, you can pick up the book again and refer to "Contents by Subjects" for techniques relating to acceptance, understanding, awareness, perspective, and self-love.

So many of the lessons I've shared in this book come from my mother, who grew up poor yet happy. She is divorced yet lives each day with joy, and she experiences anxiety and depression yet does not suffer. My mother is my best teacher, and her guidance comes neither from books nor education but from the way she lives her own life. Not only does she show that it is entirely possible to be happy, always, her approach to happiness has always been practical and extremely applicable. It is with this same approach that I've written this book, and I hope that you enjoy reading in a way that uplifts you and empowers you to live each day with joy and no regrets, no matter what comes your way. Be happy, always!

Lots of love,

Xandria

CHAPTER ONE

Understanding Happiness and Unhappiness

LIFE IS EITHER A CELEBRATION OR A LESSON

<Perspective>

My husband, Yuri, likes to say that life is either a celebration or a lesson. I think that this is one of the best philosophies, because then we can truly see life as the gift that it is.

Yuri and I have been married since 2010, and we used to argue so much in those first few years. At the time, we didn't know that it was possible to disagree without arguing. We knew that it was common for couples to argue, so we honestly thought that having arguments in a relationship was normal, even healthy.

In a way, we weren't unhappy with each other. We were unhappy with the problems; the frustrations we felt toward each other indicated that we must have felt that the other person was the source of the problems. There were differences that created friction every time we tried to talk about issues that arose.

It was only when Yuri and I started to see our disagreements as *opportunities* to learn more about each other that the way we communicated changed. We stopped fighting when we viewed the differences not as *problems*, but as welcome opportunities to learn more about each other.

Not fighting doesn't mean we have no problems in our relationship. It means that we can actually talk about what is wrong without accusing the other person of being at fault.

When things are going well in our relationship, it is a celebration. When things aren't going well in our relationship, it is a lesson. Either way, we win. This small but subtle shift in perspective gave our relationship a solid foundation on which to base our work—because we stopped feeling frustrated when we were unhappy, and we started to instead see our disagreements as a way to help us learn more about ourselves and about each other.

This perspective applies to everything in life.

We all know that life is never perfect. To be born into this world, to be alive, is to experience challenges and difficulties. We know this, yet we often despair when life isn't going well.

We know that people are not perfect, that to be human is to err. Yet when people behave badly and show us their imperfections, we can get really upset.

When we really think about it, we start to wonder what it is that causes us so much unhappiness. Is it people? Is it the circumstances? Or is it our reluctance to accept the reality of what being alive means?

If we can accept that life is either a celebration or a lesson, then our perspective toward our personal challenges and difficulties will shift. This doesn't mean that we will never feel sad or upset, it means that when we do have problems, we are able to see them as opportunities to learn something valuable about ourselves.

When I was producing and hosting on a radio station, I would often come home really upset from the challenges that I was facing with the people at work. One day, Yuri said to me, "Didn't you say that one of your goals in life is to grow as person? Well, the universe must have heard you, because it has given you this challenge to learn from and grow."

That stopped all my moaning, complaining, and feelings of self-pity. It got me thinking. He was right—if life does not present us with challenges, how are we to grow as people? If we are never tested, how will we know the level of our strength?

My challenges with my co-workers didn't disappear overnight, but my perspective on those challenges completely changed. My problems were not problems anymore, they turned into welcome challenges. The situation had not changed, yet my *feelings* toward the situation had shifted, which made such a difference in my happiness.

When I look back at that challenging time in my life, I am in awe of how much it taught me about patience and understanding. I learned how to recognize my ego and to practice the art of letting go. Of course, when I was going through the difficult times, it didn't *feel* like the situation was something to appreciate. However, when the circumstances had passed—as all things do, the good and the bad—I told my mom, "Gosh, these are lessons that I would have *paid* to learn!"

When things are going smoothly in our lives, it is a celebration. When challenges present themselves in the form of either people or our circumstances, it is an opportunity to learn. Either way, we win.

This means that we are in acceptance of what is happening— not because we have no choice, but because we know it truly benefits us.

Life is either a celebration or a lesson. This worldview provides a solid foundation for every challenge that comes our way because it encourages acceptance. Acceptance is the foundation of our happiness, much like how a structure with a solid foundation will stand strong through the worst storms. Without acceptance as our solid foundation, it will be very difficult for us to be happy or fulfilled no matter what we do or how hard we try to make things better on the surface—we will be too consumed by what is happening to us to focus our attention on resolving our problems and moving forward.

Acceptance helps us face what is happening in our lives without wishing for reality to be different. It helps us acknowledge what we feel without wishing that we were feeling something else. It is knowing that while we cannot change the reality, we have complete power over how we respond to our challenges. Acceptance helps ground us to weather the storms that will inevitably come our way.

Where there is acceptance, there is a lack of suffering. And ultimately, *happiness* is simply a lack of suffering.

PEOPLE CAN CAUSE US PAIN, BUT WE CAN CHOOSE NOT TO SUFFER

<Acceptance>

After thirty-two years of marriage, my dad came home one day and told my mom that he had fallen in love with someone else.

It was close to midnight, and I was packing for a friend's wedding in Hong Kong when my mom called with the news. There are some moments in life you remember vividly, and this was one of them. My mom said, "Girl, your dad just told me that he's met someone and he wants to be with her."

We didn't see it coming, especially my brother. My parents had had a wonderful relationship when we were growing up, and we had always been a close-knit family. It wasn't a case of pretending that everything was smooth on the surface while things were falling apart. My parents were genuine partners in every aspect of life, raising us as a team and even running a catering business and a bookshop together for more than two decades.

Yet, when we thought about it, we could see that it wasn't out of the blue. After my dad had decided to sell his business and retire, he started to be discontented with life. Perhaps he felt a loss of a sense of identity, and it became harder for him to feel fulfilled and significant without a clear purpose. My mom had a career, and my brother and I were grown and didn't need him like we had when we were younger.

It had been hard for my dad to be happy. So although his affair took us by surprise, it wasn't completely surprising.

The night my dad made his announcement, I told my friend I couldn't make it to her wedding after all. Instead of driving to the airport, I went to my parents' house. Emotions were running high, and there certainly were a lot of tears, but it wasn't frantic or loud. We were talking openly and trying to process and understand what had happened and why. My dad earnestly told us that the reason he hadn't told the family sooner was because he wasn't sure if the relationship with the other woman would work out long term.

My brother Sean, who was twenty at the time, was still attending university. It was the most upset—and probably most expressive— I've ever seen him. He didn't shout or raise his voice, but with a quiet rage he told my dad, "You punished me for telling a lie when I was young. You made me promise not to lie ever again. And now...you do *this*."

By *this*, my brother meant my dad hiding his intentions about his trip overseas, pretending it was for business, yet all the while making arrangements to meet a woman whom he had been courting over the internet. We were all blindsided by my father's affair, but in a way, I think it was my brother who felt the most betrayed.

Clearly, my dad had done something that had a chain-reaction effect on the rest of his family, but I don't think he comprehended how he had just upended my brother's world.

I was older, and in the last few years before his affair, my mother and I had had many conversations with my dad about happiness, mindset, and gratitude in hopes of lifting him up from his discontentment. So in a way, it was easier for me to see my dad as a person, separate from his role as a father.

But my brother had always viewed our dad as a *father*—strong and always right. And so for him, the very foundation on which his world rested was suddenly no longer solid. When you feel like your father has betrayed you, your world changes. I think my brother lost the last of the innocence that kids have about the world being black and white. He grew up overnight.

At times like these, families can fall apart and there can be a great deal of anger and blame. However, this didn't happen for one single reason—my mom. Where my dad shocked us with his news, my mom blew us away with her grace.

My mom responded to the entire divorce in a way that made us respect her on a whole new level. Some of us lose our minds when we get upset and lose sight of what's important to us—but not my mom. She was definitely hurt and upset, but she wasn't angry or vindictive. She never once thought my dad was a terrible person for what he'd done. For my mom, what my dad did was painful, but she believed that only *she* could choose whether or not to suffer. To her, being angry would be to suffer, and she didn't want that. Her priority was her happiness and the happiness of her children—not what my dad did or didn't do.

We'd known our mom to be kind and extremely wise from the way she raised us. People usually show us who they are when they have to go through a difficult time, and through our parents' divorce, we kept seeing evidence of our mom's kindness and wisdom.

When my dad was in the process of moving out from our house, my mom *helped him pack*. My dad wanted more time, but my mom was very firm about him moving out within a week, and she saw that the process would go more quickly if she helped with the packing.

My brother and I watched with complete fascination—and a little dismay—as she packed my dad's clothes neatly into boxes, even going so far as to label them. My brother objected to my dad taking anything other than his clothes, but unbeknownst to us at the time, my mom had given my dad a set of kitchen utensils and cutleries for his new place. It wasn't just *one* plate and a spoon, fork, and knife—it was a set of six!—because, "What if he had guests over?" Our jaws dropped when she told us this years later.

"Even in the movies you don't see people doing that!" my brother exclaimed. At the time, we both protested that my mom was being too nice to my dad. "People usually just throw everything into garbage bags and dump them outside!" I pointed out, exasperated.

It was as if we had to *remind* my mom that she was the victim here!

And then it really hit me—*why would we want my mom to think that she was a victim, when she didn't see herself as one?*

It does not take strength to hate someone, it takes strength to be *kind* to them even when they have done you a bad turn. My mom wasn't forcing herself to be nice or kind, she has always been a nice and kind person—while my mom certainly didn't think that my dad respected her in his actions, she respected *herself* enough not to behave in a way that was beneath her standards. Just because someone had been unkind did not mean she had to *also* be unkind. My mom saw no reason to let a negative experience change her for the worse.

Through the entire divorce process, my mom wasn't controlling or suppressing her emotions. She felt all sorts of emotions, but she did the same thing she had been practicing all her life whenever she was upset—she let go of the feeling. Ever since I can remember, my mom has always been someone who believes that anger solves nothing and creates more suffering. My dad may have left, but my mom did not let that change her for the worse or make her bitter.

Often, when marriages end and one parent blames the other, it makes it very difficult for the kids to be happy because they feel like they have to be just as angry as a show of support to the injured party. But because of the classy and graceful way my mom handled my dad's affair and the divorce, my brother and I didn't see it as something negative or bad.

In fact, it was incredibly inspiring to bear witness to how my mother handled this difficult time in her life. She had always taught me to be happy, but through her own actions, I could actually *see* what non-suffering meant. From the very beginning, my mom accepted the reality of what was happening without going down the path of *"How could you?!"* or *"Why me?"* In the absence of blame or self-pity, my mom suffered very little, if at all.

My mom has shown me what it truly means to be a strong person.

People can always cause us pain, but we truly can choose not to suffer. We can value our happiness so much that even when people hurt us, we don't have to give our happiness away.

WE CAN ALWAYS CHOOSE, BUT NEVER CONTROL, OUR HAPPINESS

<Acceptance>

Most of us know that happiness goes beyond a feeling—that happiness is a choice. However, sometimes we just don't feel good despite *wanting* to make the choice to be happy. Sometimes we wake up feeling depressed or anxious, and the knowledge that happiness is a choice can make us feel even *more* depressed because we feel that we have failed in some way. We feel even more frustrated at our inability to make the choice to be happy.

But here is what is important to understand—making a choice is not as the same as having control. One of the main reasons we feel frustrated at not being able to be happy is because we think our happiness is something we can control.

The problem with trying to control our lives and how we feel is that we will rarely or never succeed, because we cannot control what happens to us, and to a great extent, we cannot control how we feel. Our emotions are tied to good news and bad news, likes and dislikes, love and pain. To say that we shouldn't feel a certain way is to deny our humanity. Every emotion we feel is part of being human. To be human with grace, we need to accept that we are full of thoughts, ideas, and emotions that make us capable of extreme greatness as well as incredible sorrow.

Life takes us where it wants to take us, and the best thing we can do for ourselves is to make the choice to influence, to steer, to drive it—but we can only do that if we're *not fighting* against our own thoughts and our emotions.

When people talk about the secret of happiness, they're not talking about how we can constantly feel pleasure and elation, but how we can be in a state of contentment and peace. To be at peace is to look all the bad things fully in the face and say, "I'm not going to fight you."

When we feel we need to protect ourselves, our instincts are always to resist. We feel that resisting means we are not giving up. But it's in fact the *opposite*—resisting what we feel makes it even harder to be happy, because we are constantly feeling guilty for feeling bad. In a way, the unwillingness to accept how we feel means we are rejecting ourselves over and over again, making it very hard for us to see the value of our lives.

This is where all of us have to know that accepting our own negativity, sadness, or depression is *not* giving up. Giving acceptance to ourselves is giving kindness. It's giving understanding. It's *not* saying, "You ruined your own life because you can't feel happy."

Acceptance is saying, "It's okay, breath by breath, you can try again tomorrow."

All of us have experienced moments of deep sadness and negativity; we have days where we feel down without any real reason why. If we can be kind to ourselves during these moments instead of being frustrated at ourselves, it's already a step forward.

What's so crucial for us to understand is that moving forward in life isn't about never taking steps backwards. Sometimes we move three steps forward and five steps back. It can be incredibly frustrating because we feel like we've tried so hard to climb up, only to slide back down again. But that's not failing, that's simply *living*.

We understand that no one is perfect, so why are we so hard on ourselves during the times when we are not perfect?

So often, we think that we must control our emotions. We must control our lives. But control is only an illusion—that's why our efforts to control almost always backfire and we end up feeling worse. In life, we cannot control how we feel or how things happen, but we have absolute power over the way we respond to them.

Choosing happiness is not about controlling our emotions—it's not suddenly going from feeling sad to feeling happy the next moment. When we choose happiness, it means we understand that the *value of our lives* is never defined by *how we feel* at that moment.

We don't look at people who are unhappy and think that their lives are worth less. Don't just practice kindness toward others, and don't learn to only love others. When we practice accepting the *entirety* of what makes us...*us*—the good times and the not-so-good times—it means we are practicing loving kindness toward ourselves.

DEPRESSION IS NOT
OUR IDENTITY

<Acceptance>

My late maternal grandmother was extremely poor, and she had to work tirelessly to feed her family of ten children. I remember my mom telling me how she grew up in a rubber plantation where she and the elder siblings would wake a few hours before sunrise and take turns accompanying my grandmother out into the rubber plantation to tap rubber. Home was tiny quarters on the plantation provided by the plantation owner.

When my mom was in high school, my maternal grandparents moved and started running a coffee shop business in the small town of Malacca, Malaysia.

My grandmother would cook and sell Chicken Rice, Economy Rice (simple fare consisting of a variety of Chinese-style dishes, perhaps better known as *"Chap Fan"*), Fried *Mee Hoon* (rice vermicelli), and *Nasi Lemak*, a fragrant rice dish cooked in coconut milk accompanied by condiments. My grandfather would make 'Bao' from scratch, a Chinese steamed pastry delicacy. He would knead the dough by hand and patiently cook the different sweet and savory fillings nestled within the delicious buns. The buns are similar to what you would find in a *Dim Sum* restaurant, but my grandfather's steaming *"Baos"* were sold to neighbors and friends, with the help of his children knocking door to door.

Home was then a small flat where all ten siblings slept on a makeshift bed made out of desks pushed together. *"You slept on a desk?"* I later asked my mom in disbelief.

It's interesting how something so hard for me to imagine was so normal for my mom. I couldn't stop thinking about how uncomfortable it must have been to use desks as beds, but it wasn't even an issue for her. The family was poor all through my mom's growing-up years, yet my mom remembers having had a really happy childhood.

Happy as they were, things were not easy, and in fact, were often extremely difficult. They were always trying to make ends meet. My late grandfather was asthmatic, and when he had an asthma attack, which was often, he couldn't go to work. My grandmother was the backbone of the family and the business, and she never took any breaks. She worked through all ten pregnancies and was always right back on her feet right after giving birth. There was no luxurious time to take a proper rest as one should after childbirth.

All this took a huge toll on my grandmother's health. She suffered from a constant stream of bodily aches and pains in her later years. She also suffered through a severe menopause, feeling listlessness and entering a deep depression.

Without knowing at the time it was menopause that was causing this discomfort, the family tried to cheer her up, taking turns to be with her so she wasn't alone and helping her to think positively. It was only later that the family learned what menopause was— thinking positively didn't really help because it wasn't her mind that was causing her to feel depressed, it was her body. The moment they understood this, they sought professional help for my grandmother.

This was when I saw what acceptance means when it comes to depression. Nobody tried to "fix" my grandmother because they didn't see her as anything that was broken. My grandmother herself didn't fight against it once she understood what it was. I know my grandmother lived with pain almost daily, either physically or psychologically, but I never once heard her complain.

Whenever we would feel sad to see her in pain, she would say, *"There's nothing to be sad about, this is part of growing old."*

My grandmother was human, so she clearly must have felt every single emotion, but whenever she experienced pain, she had always accepted it as something she had to go through as part of her life. My grandmother never went to school; she never read books or lived beyond the life she created for her family, yet she has this infinite wisdom that always came from deep within.

I don't think my grandmother actively practiced acceptance as an intentional way of doing things, it was just the kind of person she was—she didn't complain, she didn't pity herself, she wasn't pretending to be happy or sitting around wishing things were different. To her, what was happening as simply what was happening, and she took joy in the smallest things in life.

My grandmother may have suffered physically, but because she accepted her situation, she was able to go through life with peace of mind and live each day with happiness.

Later, my mom, too, went through menopause. I was staying with my mom then, so it was literally closer to home, and I could see how difficult some days were for my mom. Yet, like my grandmother, my mom was able to accept the waves of depression that came with menopause. Even now, when she has days that aren't particularly good, she just tells herself that her feelings of depression are a hormonal imbalance caused by menopause and that this is just another part of her life process.

When we think about fighting depression, fighting for survival, or fighting for happiness, it is almost instinctive to fight with a refusal to accept our circumstances. Acceptance can be seen as weak or passive, but in truth, it takes someone extremely strong to accept a situation they *cannot change* and to learn to find a way around that. A fighting spirit comes not from resistance but acceptance. This is because our fight against our negative emotions and the challenges we face isn't about crashing against the waves and going against the current—the way to fight successfully lies in the ability to accept the situation and the reality of what is happening, without the "if onlys" and "what ifs."

We might not like our reality, but we should understand that if we keep wishing that our reality was different, it doesn't mean that we're actually fighting it, it means that we're *resisting*. We cannot be focused on being strong or moving forward when we are occupied with pushing back.

My mom fought her depression, but she did it by accepting it and telling herself that it was just temporary. My mom explained to me that while she might be feeling depressed, she was not *in* depression. To her, this was a very important difference. My mom accepted her feelings of depression, but not for one second did she allow depression to be her identity.

There was no denial or resistance to how she felt during that time, and because of that, it was easier for her to see that she was *more* than her depression.

Acceptance is the best way to *win* a fight.

Winning in life isn't about achieving a goal or reaching a destination, winning in life is about having a quality of life *while* we are pursuing our goals and dreams. Our quality of life is much more linked to our peace of mind than it is to what we have or don't have.

This is the main reason why my grandmother and mother are able to feel depressed yet happy at the same time, because they see that happiness is more than a feeling, it is a state of peace and contentment. Both of these women are an inspiration, as they are an example of how we can all always *value ourselves* no matter how we feel.

IT'S OKAY TO BE NOT OKAY

<Acceptance>

When we are physically injured, everyone can see it; most people will even have sympathy for a physical injury, like when we have a broken arm or leg. But when we're mentally and emotionally hurt, it's something that people cannot see. And because of the lack of tangible evidence, it is so much harder to actually explain and justify our unhappiness, even to ourselves.

No one thinks they are "not normal" when they have a fever, yet we'll ask ourselves if we're "not normal" when we feel depressed.

One of the problems with happiness is the way we view *un*happiness. We seem to see unhappiness as "not normal." But there is no *normal* state of being—to be human is to experience *all* emotions: happiness and sadness, joy and grief.

So many of us think that when we're not happy, something is wrong. We take note of the times we feel sad, down, and depressed, and we allow these experiences and feelings to make us believe that our life isn't very valuable. We don't think it consciously, but the despair we feel comes from a sense of worthlessness, where it becomes hard to see the meaning of our lives.

We do not look down upon a child born without arms or a person who is deaf, we don't pity them or treat them with disdain; we see them as they are—human beings who can make choices about how they want to live their lives. So why would we see our own sadness or depression as a disability that is crippling us? It's just *part* of who we are. There's nothing *wrong* with us when we don't feel happy.

No matter how dark the days get, no matter how difficult it is to just get through another day, remember that you are human and that human beings have to face and resolve many issues in life. Sometimes, we have to live with the issues we cannot solve.

One thing is clear—the solutions to problems, including those of physical and mental pain, don't come from hating ourselves or hating our own lives. There is always a reason for the sadness we feel, and we need to examine the source. If it's something we can work on ourselves, then we can practice letting go and removing what is stopping us from being able to access our happiness. If it's not something we can do on our own, we can seek professional help.

When you're not feeling well, remember that you are not lacking or stupid or weak—you are human, and your mind or body is telling you it needs some help, along with a lot of understanding and loving kindness from you.

I talked about this with my mom, who faces a few health challenges in life that cause her pain and physical discomfort. Despite what she experiences, she has always been happy with her life. She faces her challenges by taking actions to put things right and not fighting the situation that already exists.

My mom is human, so there are days where she feels emotionally affected and down. Some nights, she has anxiety attacks that keep her up. When things are difficult, it is her ability to be able to experience discomfort or pain without suffering that give her the ability to be at peace and to be happy.

The choice to not suffer isn't just a feeling, it's a practice. I've seen my mom going through the different stages of acceptance over the years; it takes practice to accept, let go, and be at peace.

When we experience hardships, it doesn't matter that we can't immediately change how we feel toward them. We may go through a process of wishing that things were different, and from there, move forward with trying to accept our situation, and then one day, find ourselves able to truly be at peace with something that used to bother us. *It is as it is.*

The practice of acceptance does not start with ignoring the fact that we are unhappy, pretending that we don't feel depressed, nor with brushing away or burying all the difficult emotions we feel. In fact, it's the opposite—we can only make the choice to not suffer if we can fully acknowledge what we're feeling without denial, and most importantly, without guilt, blame, or resentment.

Having seen my grandmother and my mom go through this, it is evident that being at peace even through pain is not merely wishful thinking but a definite possibility. This always reminds me of how we all have such a huge capacity to appreciate and value our lives even when we don't feel our best.

Our lives do not become less valuable when we suffer, and this is what we need to remember on the days when it's difficult to be happy. Don't let your definition of happiness be based on the feeling you have when everything is going well and there are no problems.

The path on which life takes us is not up to us to dictate and control. Even when we take care of our health, we can still fall ill. Even when we are the nicest and kindest people we are able to be, we can still get hurt. Where there is pleasure, there is always displeasure. Where there is excitement, there is always boredom. Where there is health, there is always sooner or later illness as well. Where there is love, there is always heartbreak.

This is the way life is.

People can support us, but only we can help ourselves; and it starts with *being okay with not being okay.* When we give ourselves permission to accept the bad days, the negative days, and the depressed days...then we can truly appreciate being alive, no matter the circumstance.

WE CANNOT FIND HAPPINESS, BECAUSE IT HAS NEVER BEEN LOST

<Understanding>

When we're feeling discontented with life, we often want to "find" happiness.

This is why happiness can seem so elusive to so many of us—we're constantly seeking something that cannot be found. But how can we *find* something that's *not lost* in the first place?

We use the word *unhappy* when the feeling of happiness is absent, but what we often mean is that we're frustrated or dissatisfied or upset or lost. What's important to know is that when we feel this way, our happiness has not *disappeared*—our happiness is still right there, it's just that there are so many difficulties and challenges in life to contend with that they may become barriers that block our access to our happiness.

As human beings, it is already part of our instincts to try to be happy when we are unhappy, and this is a major reason why we automatically default to *seeking* happiness when we are unhappy.

This is why it's instinctive for us to seek external pleasure when we're feeling down, because it truly does lift us up for a while. We go away on a holiday and we feel better (until we get home). We indulge in retail therapy and we feel better (until the bill comes). We finish a pint of ice cream and we feel better (until we start to feel fat). Yet at some point, most, if not all of us, recognize that our spike in happiness is temporary, that we almost always feel the same way, if not worse, after we've indulged in the pleasures that life has to offer.

The unhappiness lingers, even after we've tried so hard to lift ourselves up. This is because the obstacles that block our access to our happiness firmly remain where they are. It's not that we're not trying to be happy, it's that our efforts are always spent trying to navigate *around* the obstacles instead of removing them from our path. We get very good at addressing the symptoms of our problems without identifying or understanding the root causes of our unhappiness.

What are the barriers between us and our happiness?

When we look on the surface, the barriers to joy are stressful work situations, painful relationships, and difficult people. But when we look beyond the surface and delve deeper, we will begin to see that it is *we ourselves* who are blocking the way to our own happiness—with our needs, fears, insecurities, resentment, anger, and all the emotions and expectations that weigh us down because we cannot let go of them. It is always what is unresolved in our hearts and minds that stops us from being able to be at peace.

This can sound like bad news, but when you think about it, it's actually a relief. Because when you know that you are the source of what is keeping you away from the happiness in your life, then you know that you are *also* the person capable of changing it.

Even though it can seem scary to take responsibility for our happiness, it's actually empowering. The power we all have over the quality of our lives is immense. Life is not what or who happens to us, it is how we *respond* to what or who happens to us, and our responses are always a *manifestation* of our own perspective, needs, and fears.

This is why when life is difficult, it doesn't help our happiness to look outside ourselves, because that leads us down the path of seeking happiness externally without understanding ourselves, which means any pleasure gained is short-lived.

Because of this, we can feel like we're constantly trying so hard to figure out ways to be happy at work and in our relationships, yet we're ending up frustrated that it's not paying off. Also, in the same way, we can feel like we're putting in so much effort to be nice and understanding yet still wind up feeling it's never enough.

This is why when we're not happy in our job, we change jobs. It's why when we're not happy in a relationship, we find a new relationship. Yet we still continue feeling unhappy. No matter how hard we try, our problems are either still there or they manifest in other ways.

It's not that we cannot change jobs or relationships—in fact, we must discern when to *exit* something that is not healthy for us—but often we don't know whether to stay or when to leave because we don't understand ourselves well enough. If we don't thoroughly understand ourselves, we will always be trying to find happiness externally.

Feeling unhappy is part of life, and when we are unhappy, it's important not to merely seek happiness but to *uncover* the layers upon layers of what is blocking our access to our happiness—and that requires us to look within.

If we don't understand ourselves, we'll keep blaming people and circumstances for causing our unhappiness, and we won't be able to truly identify the root of what is holding us back. We'll keep feeling frustrated and angry and jealous and resentful and guilty and shameful without the awareness that *we can release ourselves* from all these barriers—because the roadblocks to our happiness are internal.

If we keep looking outwards when we have problems—if we keep thinking that it is other people or the environment that are the problem—then we will find ourselves repeating the same pattern of unhappiness and discontentment over and over again. We won't be able to be happy no matter where we work or how wonderful our relationship partner is.

What helps us identify and remove the barriers to our happiness is to look within to understand *why* we are allowing people and circumstance to have such a negative impact on us. This is when our minds have the clarity to see that our reactions to people and circumstances are often driven by our insecurities, fears, needs, expectations, judgements, self-righteousness, and so much more.

If we don't recognize that our happiness has always been with us, we will end up seeking happiness in the form of emotions, and we'll try to constantly create the feeling of pleasure, euphoria, or elation. We may even search for happiness like it's a goal or something to be achieved.

Yet no matter how hard we search, if we are not willing to work on ourselves, we won't be able to access our happiness no matter where we go, whom we're with, or what we do. This is why we can have the most amazing careers and the most loving families yet feel unfulfilled in life. In life, it doesn't bode well for us to seek more happiness to *replace* the unhappiness we feel. Inner peace just doesn't work that way.

There is no antidote in the outside world for the unhappiness we feel deep within. Things will happen to us, and people will affect us, but only we have absolute power over the joy we have. This helps us understand that while things may not be our *fault,* our happiness is always our *responsibility.*

No matter who or what happens in our lives, it really helps to understand that our joy has not disappeared. The work isn't to *find* happiness, but to *remove* the barriers to being able to deal with our own suffering and unhappiness. Peace is something that only we can give ourselves.

SELF-CRITICISM IS NOT SELF-IMPROVEMENT

<Self-Love>

Looking inward to identify the barriers to our happiness isn't about beating ourselves up. Taking responsibility for our own happiness is not about blaming ourselves. It's not about willingly taking on guilt and thinking, "It's my fault!" or "I'm so stupid!" It's really important to understand that self-improvement is not self-criticism.

Taking responsibility for our own happiness is about letting go of the concept of blame altogether—both toward others and toward ourselves—because this means we truly understand and accept that our difficulties are part and parcel of being alive.

If we are critical of ourselves, it's harder for us to be honest about our needs and fears. When we receive criticism—even from ourselves—the natural reaction is defense. We *defend ourselves against ourselves* without even realizing it. What this means is that it's very easy to be in denial about where we need to improve as people because we don't feel safe enough to be honest with ourselves.

How can you feel sufficiently safe to be honest with yourself when you are always judging yourself?

This is why even when we genuinely *want* to improve ourselves, we can find it so difficult—we want to transform, yet part of us blocks it out. We are resisting change even while we are desiring change.

So criticizing ourselves only *seems* like a good tool for improvement, while it is in fact detrimental to being a better person. We can also *think* we are improving while in reality we are regressing, because our self-protective mechanism has kicked in to prevent us from seeing our own flaws.

Some of us think we are self-aware, but we are actually in denial.

Although it may seem counterintuitive, it is not self-criticism but *self-acceptance* that is key to self-improvement.

When we can accept ourselves, it means that we are not subconsciously judging ourselves or being resentful of who we are. This means we feel safe enough to *be honest and acknowledge* our shortcomings and weaknesses, and that we do not feel so guilty and ashamed that we have to block them out or make excuses for ourselves.

Self-criticism is one of the main reasons why even as we are working so hard on being happy, we still find ourselves unhappy. If we self-criticize and constantly beat ourselves up, it means we don't accept ourselves. If we don't accept ourselves, it means that we are constantly attributing blame for our unhappiness, which is as unhealthy as blaming *others* for our unhappiness.

Our lack of self-acceptance manifests in our reactions toward people—we'll constantly feel that we are lacking, and this results in always comparing ourselves to others. It's also why we can be so sensitive to what people think of us. Always subconsciously seeking acceptance from others makes it very hard for us to be at peace.

Until we stop criticizing ourselves for not being good enough, we won't understand that our happiness has never been about being good enough or perfect enough, because we have *always been enough*. To be human is to already be imperfect, which means that we are bound to experience doubts, insecurities, needs, and fears.

My husband Yuri likes to say that we are like Swiss cheese—it has plenty of holes but is perfect the way it is. I laughed when he said it, but the image holds such truth! We have to work on filling up the holes and gaps in our lives (and therefore we seek self-improvement), yet we are simultaneously also perfect the way we are (hence the self-acceptance).

If we keep creating conditions listing what we must achieve to be happy, or how we must feel to be happy, or how our life has to be for us to be happy...then we will always be at the mercy of our own discontentment.

The other thing to understand is that if we use self-criticism as a way to motivate ourselves to be better, not only will it backfire, it also means that we will likely employ the same methods on the people around us—we will think that it is a good thing to criticize those we love because it will "motivate" them to be better. Then, the same cycle of unhappiness will plague the people closest to us.

We can only access our happiness when we can recognize what holds us back or weighs us down. This requires us to first *accept* and *love* ourselves so that we can freely identify the barriers to our happiness without guilt and shame making us resistant and defensive.

WE ARE NEVER
THE VICTIM
WHEN WE VALUE
OURSELVES

<Self-Love>

One of the essential foundations of self-love is seeing our own value and respecting ourselves.

"Love yourself" was the advice that my late grandma gave my mother when she left home at age seventeen to journey from her small hometown to the big city for a brighter future. My grandma wasn't a person who nagged at or fretted about her kids. Instead, she had a way of making them understand the enormity of her message in just a few simple words. So *love yourself* were two words that stayed with my mom as she grew into adulthood.

When I left home for the first time and went abroad to study at a university, my mom said the same thing to me: "Love yourself." I remember talking to her about what it meant. The concept of self-love was hard for me to grasp back then, but I could feel the significance of what she was trying to convey.

It wasn't until I started dating and fell in love that it really hit home how valuable that advice was. It almost sounds too simple— love yourself, but it means *so much*. Loving yourself means that you never attach your self-worth to whether or not someone loves you.

When my dad told my mom that he was having an affair and wanted to be with someone else, my mom felt a torrent of emotions. But there was one thing she did not feel—she *did not* feel that my dad had fallen in love with someone else because she wasn't good enough.

We often wonder: *how* do you love yourself? We understand the concept of self-love, yet when it comes down to it, what does it really mean?

My mom taught me self-love, and when I watched my mom's reactions and decisions through her divorce process, I could *see* what the practice of self-love meant. I could see my mom's sadness and pain, yet *not once* did she blame herself or beat herself up wondering if she had been a "good enough wife." She knew that she had done her best for the relationship as a wife, as a best friend, and as a woman. My mom didn't blame my dad because she didn't attach *her own value* as a person to his decision to leave.

My mom respected herself enough to not see herself as a victim, so she simply wasn't one. The truth is, people can only victimize us in this way when we give them responsibility for our happiness. It is easy to feel lost when we feel like the people we love don't value us, but it is so important to know that the *value of who we are as people* does not diminish based on how other people see us. Don't let your worthiness be determined by how someone treats you.

When we are in relationships, our happiness is still and will always be our own responsibility. And if your happiness is your own responsibility, then no one can ever make you feel diminished or unworthy. And that is self-love and self-respect.

NOBODY CAN MAKE US
HAPPY OR UNHAPPY

<Perspective>

One of the main reasons why we unconsciously give our happiness away so easily to others is because we think that other people make us happy or unhappy.

When we go into a relationship or marry someone, it is because the person brings so much joy into our lives. When we fall in love, every other kind of happiness that we've ever felt can pale in comparison; so much so that it's natural for us to settle on this one thought: *this person makes me happy.*

But that isn't true.

It is *you* who made yourself happy—you made the choice to allow yourself to open up to someone incredible. You made the decision to commit to someone to whom you feel extremely connected. You made the choice to stick around and to hang in there through all the challenges and difficulties.

Nobody can *make* us happy, we have always been the ones who have brought happiness into our own lives.

If you're feeling happy because you have great friends, it's because you have chosen to surround yourself with genuine, generous, and loving people. If you're feeling happy because you have a great family, it's because you have chosen to be consciously grateful for them.

Similarly, nobody can make us *un*happy. No wife, no husband, no boyfriend or girlfriend, lovers or exes, family or friends can *make* us unhappy—we have always been the only ones who can cause our own suffering and our own unhappiness, because it is always our *response* to the circumstances that determines whether we are happy or unhappy.

It's never what happens or who happened, but how we handle it. It is also not whom we have or don't have in our lives, because we cannot have a healthy relationship until we know that our happiness cannot be given to us by someone else.

We don't expect people to lose weight for us, so why would we expect people to make us happy? We have to do that ourselves.

This is a perspective that my dad has never been able to truly understand. So much of his unhappiness lies in him being constantly at the mercy of people and circumstances—the smallest thing can make him angry, put him in a bad mood, and affect his entire day, if not his entire week.

Most of us don't consciously think, "I blame the weather, the traffic, the waiter, that stupid person, my partner, and/or my boss," but that *is* essentially what we're doing when we have a tendency to be easily upset by people and circumstances.

When our thoughts carry us in a direction of blame, it is very easy to feel sorry for ourselves because we feel like people and things are always creating unhappiness in our lives. But our happiness is not in the hands of people and circumstances, it is *inside* of us.

As long as we are seeking happiness externally instead of cultivating it internally, it is likely it will be very hard for us to live with gratitude, because every time we feel grateful about something, we will find fault with a dozen other things.

Nobody can make us happy or unhappy, but *we* can *always* make ourselves happy.

CHAPTER TWO

Fulfilment in Love and Relationships

UNDERSTAND THE RELATIONSHIP YOU HAVE WITH YOURSELF

<Understanding>

One of our deepest needs for happiness, or even for survival, revolves strongly around our connections and relationships with people. However, it is often our connections and relationships with people that cause us the most problems and bring us the most unhappiness. The one thing we need the most is also the one thing that challenges us the most. It would be very ironic if it didn't make so much sense—where there is comfort, there is also challenge. The yin and yang of life is what creates balance, and to deny one by craving more of the other only serves to make us miserable.

Our quality of life is greatly impacted by the quality of our relationships with people, so if we don't cultivate the skills of how to navigate through the difficult aspects of interacting with others, we will often feel very unhappy.

This is why we can have so much going for us yet feel so angry or frustrated most of the time. We can have an amazing career we know we're lucky to have, yet go to work in a bad mood because we can't get along with a colleague or with our boss. We can have a steady relationship we value, yet still feel resentful of our partner and what he or she isn't contributing to the relationship. We can have a beautiful family we love, yet spend most of our time at home, impatient and short-tempered.

Life is strange in the way that we can see how much we have yet still not feel content. If this isn't addressed, we will go through life chalking up many regrets along the way. Many of us are aware of this already, but we don't know how to resolve the feelings of discontentment within us.

This is why I find it so important to learn how to build positive relationships with others, because it is the people around us who impact our happiness the most. Much of our dissatisfaction with life comes from dissatisfying interactions and relationships.

When it comes to relationships with people, it isn't about making people happy or blaming and accusing those who make you unhappy—it's about understanding your relationship with yourself.

It isn't until we examine what our needs and fears are that we understand why we have an aversion to certain behaviors, or why we gravitate toward certain relationships, or why we put up a wall to protect ourselves.

It isn't until we know what our ideals and expectations are that we understand why some people affect us more deeply than others, or why we might have a really strong negative reaction when people disagree with us.

We can be incredibly good with the day-to-day things of living, from feeding ourselves and our families to managing teams of people and putting out fires at work. This is partly because we spend years in school preparing ourselves for our careers, so as adults, a huge part of our brain space is dedicated to thinking about how to do or fix something. However, to be truly happy, we also need to learn to be aware of why we think the thoughts we do, why we want the things we want, and why we get upset over certain things. It is when we understand ourselves that we can stop outsourcing our happiness away so easily to other people.

Problems and challenges are inevitable in our relationships— pain and hurt are part of human interaction—but it is how we respond to them that determines how happy we are. To resolve problems in our relationships with people, we have to learn how to communicate. The hardest part about communicating with people is learning not to react negatively when we disagree—it's hard to not feel defensive, judged, resentful, or attacked in a difficult conversation. This makes it hard for us to take the next step forward or to make decisions that can help us and not hurt us further. This is why before we can even begin to understand someone else, we have to first understand ourselves.

What are your expectations and judgements of other people? What are your triggers and sensitivities? What are your insecurities, fears, and needs?

To understand ourselves is to understand people better. This is the most crucial step of communication, whether in our romantic relationships, with our family members, or even with difficult clients, colleagues, and customers.

When we face challenges in our relationships with people, the work is not up to *them*—it is up to us to build our self-awareness and emotional maturity so that we can *respond* to these relationship challenges in a way that brings us more happiness and less suffering. As the next two chapters of this book address how we relate with people, it is best to read them sequentially. The next chapter examines our expectations, needs, and fears so that we will be able to communicate openly and build amazing relationships with the people we love.

YOUR NORMAL IS NOT THE UNIVERSAL NORMAL

<Perspective>

Part 1

PERSPECTIVE

Is life difficult? Or is it that the people in our lives make life difficult? The answer is almost always the latter, until we realize that this is not true either—it is *our expectations* of how people should be that make our lives difficult.

We all have our values, beliefs, principles, and ethics that we hold true, and they form the standards that guide our lives. We all think that our standards are good; that's why we subscribe to them. This is why it's easy to fall into thinking that our own standards are the *universal* standard—"Kind people will behave this way," or "Generous people will do that."

This is when we impose our definitions of what is "good" on people without realizing that we are projecting our expectations upon them. When people—strangers, colleagues, friends, and especially family—behave in ways that are different from our standards, we get upset because we genuinely don't see why they wouldn't embrace something that makes so much sense (to us).

However, we forget that what makes sense to one person may not make sense to another person. When we think that someone "has no common sense," we usually get frustrated at the person. However, how can a different person with a different background and a different personality have the exact same "normal" as we do? Common sense is not common precisely because what is common to me may not be common to you. To expect otherwise is to cause our own suffering.

The guiding principles we believe in drive how we conduct our lives, how we treat others, how professional we are at work, and how we love; and we tend to hold others to the same benchmarks. This is why it's very instinctive for us to think, *"If you love me, you would know this"* or *"Geez, if I were him, I wouldn't have done that!"* because we always compare others to what *we* ourselves would or wouldn't do.

So much of our misery and suffering comes from how we insist the world should be. If you think about it, we only get upset at someone who is behaving in a way that we wouldn't behave. *"He's so unkind!"* (I am a kind person.) *"How could she have done that?!"* (I would have the sense not to do that.)

Yet if you ask yourself about whether it's logical to expect people to do what you would do, to think the way you would think, and to behave as you would behave…you'd see that there is little possibility that over seven billion people in this world can be like you; which means that it is even more illogical to get upset when we meet people who are *not* like us.

Part 2

PERSPECTIVE

We all know that everyone is different. Why then, do we get so angry or experience such disbelief when people behave differently than ourselves?

The answer lies in how we perceive people and the world. Based on the fact that we all exist as human beings in the same universe, most of us subconsciously perceive that every human being is sharing the same reality and adhering to the same rules.

This means that, in our minds, we see ourselves as individuals living in one giant house, under the same roof. Refer to *The Expectation Circle 1: What we subconsciously assume.*

Reality

You

John   Mary

Ken   Sam

Everyone in this world

The Expectation Circle 1: What we subconsciously assume

This is why, even as we say we understand that people are different, we *still* get upset when we experience how different people are. It is because we feel like they are exhibiting behaviors that are not in line with the "house rules and standards"!

While it is true that we all live in the same universe, what is also true is this: Each individual human being has their own thoughts. Only we can experience our thoughts, so in a way, our thoughts create our own reality. Which means, there isn't *one giant* reality where seven billion of us all coexist together—what is more accurate is that there are close to seven billion *different realities* in this universe. It's like how every single person is living in their own house with their own rules.

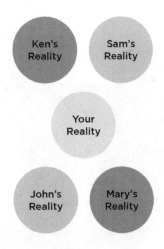

The Expectation Circle 1.1: What is more accurate

In *my* reality, the rules and what is considered normal might be the exact opposite of your rules and what you consider normal in your reality. This is why when we think someone *should* or *shouldn't* do something, it's incredibly foolish, because it indicates that we think that our normal is more normal than someone else's normal, not understanding that in their reality, we are the ones who are abnormal.

Why are we drawn to certain people, and why do we get along with them so well? The easy answer is that it's because we have many things in common. But when we examine it more closely, it is because the rules in their reality are similar to those in ours.

You, your family members, and your best friends share many similar values and perspectives such as integrity, kindness, and respect, and this is where a big part of their reality overlaps with yours. The parts that overlap are where we feel in sync with someone—"Yeah, this person gets me."

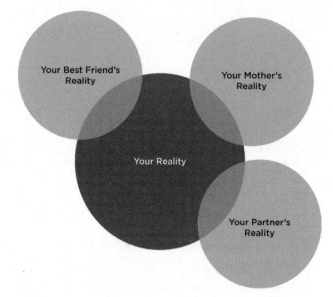

The Expectation Circle 1.2: Your circle of influence

The thing is, no single human reality ever completely overlaps that of another, because no two people are exactly the same. Even siblings or other family members who share vastly similar ideals, values, and beliefs have parts of their realities that don't intersect. It is these nonintersecting parts of personal realities that cause disagreements and arguments.

A big part of why we fall in love with someone is because the person's reality overlaps with ours. This is where we feel the most comforted, loved, safe, and happy. However, even when two people are in love, there are parts of their realities that don't overlap—this is why we can have such explosive fights with a partner and get so upset when they don't understand and don't agree with us.

Now, think of the people with whom you don't get along—people who you think have no common sense or whose behavior you do not respect. These are people whose realities have no overlap with yours. They are so different from us, they are like aliens! These are the people who we frustratingly think must be from another planet. This is where thoughts and accusations like, "I can't believe you said that!" or "How could you do this?!" often surface in a communication, creating a downward spiral that is fueled by angry disbelief.

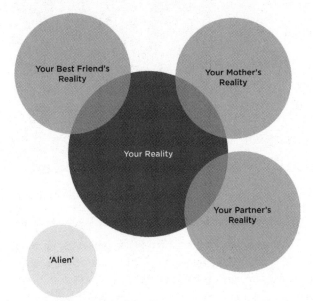

Your Best Friend's Reality

Your Mother's Reality

Your Reality

Your Partner's Reality

'Alien'

The Expectation Circle 1.3: Your relationship with people

And guess what? From the alien's point of view...*you* are the alien. Because in their reality, they also have families and friends who overlap with their reality, so to this other person, *you* are the one who is absolutely foreign.

It is often our disbelief at another person's words and actions that makes us angry, but when we understand that our normal is not someone else's normal, it is easier for us to see how it is completely possible (and only logical!) for another human being not to see our point and vice versa.

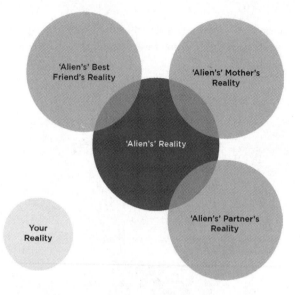

The Expectation Circle 1.4: The alien's point of view

So much of what blocks the way to our happiness is born out of our expectations of people. One of the main reasons why we are negatively affected by others is because we think they are not behaving as we think they should. It is this thinking that causes our suffering, rather than those other people causing our unhappiness.

The path to happiness lies in not forgetting that our beliefs, values, principles, and opinions are *our own* guiding principles, meant to guide us in our lives. They are not there for us to use to judge and become upset at those who have a differing or opposite way of thinking and living. There is no "should" in the way people are. There is only how we want to live our lives.

My husband likes to say, "Strong beliefs held loosely," and I think that it's a wonderful way of living life: with a strong foundation of beliefs that are not held so tightly that we become unable to see anything else.

OUR EXPECTATIONS ARE OUR STANDARDS IMPOSED UPON SOMEONE ELSE

<Understanding>

Our expectations of people are not bad, they are simply part of how human beings instinctively operate. It is natural for us to react badly against people who go against what we believe to be the right way of doing things. However, what is *instinctive* for us to experience isn't necessarily what is *healthy* for us to experience.

When it comes to relationships, our expectations are almost always well-intentioned. We think that having expectations in a relationship is good, for without expectations, we will have no standards and the relationship will not improve.

This is absolutely not true.

We can have standards without expectations. Having standards is internal—it's our own guiding principles. Having expectations, on the other hand, is external—it's wanting other people to see and do things the way we do and getting upset when they don't.

Expectations manifest when we impose our standards on the people around us. We often do this with good intentions—we genuinely believe that the person should adopt what we believe because it's a better standard compared to theirs.

However, having expectations isn't a suitable tool to use to help a relationship improve. In fact, the opposite happens and the relationship deteriorates.

In the early stages of my relationship with my husband Yuri, I had many, many expectations of him that I thought were good. I was even proud to have them, because I thought they signified that I had high standards—that I had a good code by which to live. I used to think, "I'm not asking anything of you that *I* wouldn't ask of myself," or "I'm not asking anything of you that isn't *normal.*"

Similarly, Yuri, too, had expectations of me and his own ideas of what a relationship should be, especially after we got married.

This was why the first three years of our marriage were incredibly tumultuous. We both had a lot of expectations of each other that we brought into the relationship, but we didn't question *why* we had those expectations. We just wanted each other to be a certain way—I wanted Yuri to be more helpful, he wanted me to be more giving—and even though we talked about it a million times, we still didn't receive what we wanted. We felt hurt because we felt like it was a sign that the other person didn't care enough.

At that time, we didn't know our expectations of each other were the root of our problems. We were just unhappy with each other, and quiet resentment started to grow. Resentment wasn't something we addressed, it was just there—running under the surface all the time and reflected in the arguments we had.

We loved each other, but we didn't feel loved. Even when one party was giving what was expected of them, it was done with defensiveness and resistance. It wasn't until we were able to let go of our expectations of each other that our relationship started changing for the better, because we could finally communicate with each other without arguing.

ARE YOUR EXPECTATIONS HELPING OR SABOTAGING YOU?

<Awareness>

To let go of our expectations, we have to first understand why our expectations are doing us such a disservice.

"Expectations" is just a word, but it is what the word represents that causes problems. Expectations almost always carry the concept of "should" in our minds, which brings with it furious thoughts of unfairness and indignation. When we think something is unfair or "should be different," we think we have a *right* to feel upset, so it drives us to hold on even tighter to all the negative emotions that don't serve us.

Imagine that there is no "should" in your vocabulary. If someone were to do something you don't understand, that would just be a fact. Your train of thought would be, "He doesn't understand" rather than *"But he doesn't understand!"* which implies that he *should* understand. In both trains of thought, the situation remains exactly the same—the person doesn't understand. However, the second thought (*"But he doesn't understand!"*) changes the way we *feel* about the situation or the person—we are more upset and less able to communicate effectively.

Being calm and not getting upset doesn't mean that we become doormats and let people walk all over us—it means that we are able to go through undesirable situations without our emotions affecting us so badly that it stops us from effectively addressing those situations.

People can certainly be wrong, and we must take action to solve problems, but our concept of how *people should be* can truly hamper our ability to think clearly and communicate effectively. Expectations sabotage us because instead of addressing the problem, we are addressing our emotions. It's almost like expectations blind us to solutions to a problem because our minds are too focused on what the situation *should be* and getting upset over how someone *should* behave.

At some point in our lives, it helps to ask ourselves what our expectations of people are really doing for us. What do you gain from your expectations of people? What do you lose due to your expectations of people?

Often, we gain righteous anger from our expectations of people and we lose our peace of mind due to our expectations of people.

In my relationship with Yuri, I used to experience frustration over the concept: *"Why aren't you more helpful?"* I would always feel so hurt whenever he didn't immediately offer to help me with simple things like carrying the shopping bags or when he seemed reluctant to lend his time to help me with work or to fix something. In *my* reality, it was a *normal* thing to expect that a person who loves you would not only volunteer to help, they would *happily* help. That's what *I* would do.

It was only after a few years into our relationship that I realized that:

a.   I was subconsciously comparing what he was doing to what I would do if I were him, which was why I always arrived at the conclusion that his not meeting my expectation must be because he didn't *care* enough; and

b.   My expectation of *"If people love you, they will unquestionably and happily want to help you"* is a direct manifestation of my upbringing. I realized that it was because while I was growing up, my parents had helped me so much in my life that to me, it was *normal* to want to do things for the people you love.

Similarly, Yuri, too, felt unhappy when certain aspects of his ideals weren't fulfilled; and he had his own discoveries and work to do when it came to his expectations of me as a partner.

All along, our unhappiness with each other was because we had all these ideas of how a marriage was supposed to be. Even though we were not consciously doing it, we were always measuring each other against some kind of standard, which is where all expectations were born.

Without expectations, we see someone for who they are—in all their flawed imperfection—without judgement. It doesn't mean we have to agree with them, it doesn't even mean we understand them, it just means we are not upset at them, which allows us to communicate better.

When you have a relationship with someone, it's often impossible to say who is right and who is wrong, or whose standard works better or who should adjust or change. We all have needs, fears, desires, and preferences, and the best we can do is to take responsibility for them as our personal preferences instead of imposing them onto our partner under the belief that our expectations are universal standards.

When we understand that other people's realities are different from our own, then we know that it is entirely possible to *talk* about something that we think is wrong without *accusing* the other person of being wrong.

This is the very foundation of good communication—if we cannot talk to someone without getting upset, then we will be really lousy at communicating with people even if we have intelligent points to make. Intelligence is not wisdom. Letting go of expectations, and therefore, letting go of the concept of "should," helps us let go of righteous anger, which makes it much easier to verbalize our thoughts.

Don't let your expectations sabotage your relationship and your happiness.

DON'T LET RESENTMENT EAT AWAY AT YOUR RELATIONSHIP

<Awareness>

All of us communicate using much more than just what we say or hear. Even without words, we are always communicating through the energy and vibe we bring to a space, and these are a direct manifestation of our thoughts. If we have expectations, it's no use *saying* we don't have them, because our thoughts always manifest in a vibration that can be felt by the other person.

When we have expectations of how our partner should be, our partner will *feel* like they're constantly being measured according to some sort of benchmark or ideal. As a result, they will feel judged. When they feel judged, it will cause them to feel resentful. We, in turn, can feel their resentment and resistance, and we will feel more and more frustrated about why it is becoming so much more difficult to be happy together.

This is why we can love someone so deeply and do so much for them, *yet* our relationships don't improve, because no matter how much we love someone, as long as we are holding onto our expectations, the judgement, resentment, and resistance going both ways can always be felt in a relationship.

This is why even when someone *says* "sorry" to you, you may get even more upset because you *feel* like they are holding onto resistance about the thing for which they are apologizing, and that makes you feel like their apology is not sincere. It is why you can keep *telling* someone you love them without your beloved feeling happy about it, because while you are expressing your love, they can also feel the underlying resentment you still have simmering away.

This is due to the fact that we nonverbally communicate our expectations, judgements, resentment, and resistance more loudly than the words we say out loud. We can *feel* the unhappiness our partner has toward us and vice versa—it's why both parties become more defensive and less willing to give.

This rings true in any kind of relationship, be it a relationship with a partner, family members, or our colleagues at work. It is the reason why we can put so much effort into being nice to someone—even sacrificing for the person—yet not see any improvement in the relationship. When resentment is present, no matter how hard we try, things deteriorate instead of improve.

In the first few years of my marriage with Yuri, the resentments we both carried showed up through small, everyday things, and when we tried to talk about it, we couldn't do it without arguing. It was why we could spend hours talking yet not really ever progress very far.

You can love someone, but they may not feel loved because they can feel your disapproval and judgement. This was the reason why Yuri and I didn't feel like we were supported or loved—we could also feel the underlying vibe of disapproval when one person didn't measure up to what the other one expected. Even though we didn't intentionally set out to make the other person feel like they weren't good enough, that feeling was what naturally brought up a reaction of resentment. Expectations lead to resentment, and resentment always leads to judgement.

Love is essential in a relationship, but no matter how much we love someone, it will be difficult to have a happy relationship if we have expectations evoking resentment that eats away at the love.

TO TALK INSTEAD OF ARGUE, BE CURIOUS INSTEAD OF ACCUSATORY

<Understanding>

One of my good friends, Mark, met the love of his life in London. Mark is Malaysian, and Sarah is Scottish. They have very similar values in life, which serves as a wonderful foundation for their relationship, but as far as background and culture go, they are as different as can be. As you can imagine, miscommunication and misunderstandings are hard to avoid.

Although Mark has been living in the UK for more than a decade, he is still very Asian in his beliefs, preferences, and habits, while Sarah is very Western in hers. For example, Mark gave Sarah all sorts of advice from the moment they started seriously dating. He would say what he thought she should or shouldn't do, as well as what was or wasn't a good idea in his opinion.

"The advice thing was really hard to get my head around, especially at the beginning!" Sarah told me when I asked her about it. "In my culture, as well as in my family, as an adult, people don't give unsolicited advice unless you're about to make some sort of very serious mistake that will cause huge problems!"

Sarah couldn't figure it out at first. Was Mark offering advice because he was pushy? Was it because he felt she wasn't capable enough to think for herself?

Meanwhile, Mark couldn't figure out why Sarah would get so defensive or upset every time he tried to offer advice. He felt like she didn't appreciate his efforts and support. It wasn't until many heated conversations later that they each finally started to understand where the other was coming from.

"For Mark, he was giving advice to show that he cared, loved me, and wanted to help me find the best possible solution or conclusion. What I was *hearing* when he gave me advice was the implication that I was about to make such a big *mistake* that he had to intervene," Sarah explained.

In the Asian culture, there *is* a tendency for family to poke their noses into each other's affairs, and people generally perceive it as a reflection of love and caring. You'd always hear aunties saying, *"Eat this, it's good for you! You're too skinny, you should eat more!"* or *"You're getting fat, cut down!"* In a Western context, this can be seen as disrespect or distrust.

Now that he's aware of this, Mark consciously tries to offer less advice, because he really *does* trust and respect Sarah's judgement. "But when he does say something," she tells me, "I try to take it in the spirit that it is intended and not be defensive."

Mark shared his thoughts too. "Just putting it out there—some people are generally just more comfortable with receiving advice than others. So I'm not sure if it's purely a cultural difference or perhaps just a personal preference."

That's a good point. Race and culture aside, Mark and Sarah also had *family* conditioning that led to different expectations of what it means to convey love. Sarah's family, and her dad in particular, had encouraged her to think for herself. They were always there to help when she needed it, but she grew up feeling that her parents trusted her capabilities and skills to figure out how to solve her own problems.

Mark has been giving advice to his brothers for as long as he can remember, and it was always welcomed and appreciated. He felt his brothers trusted him when he gave advice.

When you factor in the intricacies of family culture, they both had very many different expectations of what trust, support, and love mean.

According to Sarah, this was just one of the many things they had to adjust to in their relationship. They candidly shared, "It will probably always be something that we have to work at. But being able to talk about it and understand that things sometimes don't translate the way we expect them to has been really helpful."

Mark and Sarah's very obvious cultural differences may easily lead to misunderstandings, but it can also lead to easier understanding. Because they look so different, they are constantly *reminded* that they are indeed very different people who have to work hard at understanding each other. Their differences are so obvious that it's also more obvious that they need to communicate when upset, instead of just continuing to feel hurt, frustrated, or resentful. When one person does something and it upsets the other, they don't automatically assume that it's because he or she doesn't care.

So in a way, it helps their communication because they are more mindful about trying not to take things personally, and most of all, being *curious* instead *accusatory*. The perspective is different, and therefore, so is their approach to communication. There are fewer expectations and judgements and less resentment, and more effort toward seeking to understand.

What about when we are dating someone from a very similar background, culture, and race? When someone *looks* and seems very similar to us on the surface, it is very easy to forget that the person is a completely different individual, with a completely different "normal" than ourselves. However, when we fall in love with someone, it is almost instinctive to expect our partner to embody the very same principles, beliefs, and standards that we assume are common sense. This is why when our partner does something that we think is not acceptable, we become really upset, because we genuinely expect them to know better.

However, based on our *conditioning*, we all define responsibility, ambition, kindness, generosity, consideration, respect, manners, and security in a certain manner and from a certain perspective. Just like Mark and Sarah's differing family cultures, every person we come across also has their own thoughts, beliefs, preferences, and habits that have been influenced and shaped by their experiences growing up.

So when we are hurt by our partner, what really helps us is to remember that even though it *feels* personal, we don't have to take it personally. This puts us in a better frame of mind to communicate, ask questions, and listen so that we can truly understand where our partner is coming from instead of measuring them against our own benchmarks of trust, support, and love.

ARE YOUR SUBCONSCIOUS EXPECTATIONS HURTING YOUR RELATIONSHIP?

<Awareness>

Most of us learn what "love" is (and is not) through observing our parents' relationship and from absorbing society's cues from books and movies, and all of these influences merge into subconscious expectations for our own relationships. It's subconscious because at the outset, we tend to just see them as "good standards," "what is normal," or "how love should be."

Sometimes, we expect things from people because our families expect the same things from us. Sometimes, we judge people because that's how our families judge people.

As we grow older, it can be very interesting to discover that what we thought were our own opinions and preferences were actually other people's opinions and preferences that we adopted as our own.

This awareness can vastly improve our lives and our relationships. You and your partner can create your own definition of normal based on what you both want and what works for *your* relationship—not what relationships *should be*, but what *works for you both*.

People can always give you advice, and your parents may have their own way of conducting their relationship, but for you to be happy in yours, you have to question why you want certain things done a certain way—perhaps it isn't as important as you *thought* it was, and your need was just a habit that came from your family culture instead of your own personal preference.

For example, if your mom used to tell you off for chewing loudly, you might feel irritated whenever your partner eats loudly. But does it really bother you, or does it bother you because it's a habit that bothered your mom? Is your partner really rude, or have you have associated eating loudly with rudeness? Is your partner actually loud, or are you more sensitive because it's become your habit to make an effort to eat very quietly?

You might discover that hey, your partner's eating habits don't actually bother you! Or maybe you might find that it really does bother you, and then you can communicate *why* you have this preference instead of continually telling your partner not to do it "because it's rude."

This is such a small thing—the way someone eats—but in real life, there are a million small things that our partners do or don't do that irritate, frustrate, hurt, and anger us.

I remember being really upset when Yuri would hesitate or seem reluctant during the times when I asked him to pick me up from a location that was out of his way, or to drive me to the airport. My immediate thoughts were: wasn't it absolutely normal that if you loved someone, you would happily pick them up when they asked?

This was when I realized that in my family, my family would chauffeur each other around whenever we needed a ride, even if it was out of the way. That's how we grew up, so that's how we interpreted care, concern, and love. To me, it was *normal* to happily help family out in any way we could.

It was such a small thing, yet it showed me that my expectations of my partner were incredibly linked to how my family showed each other support and care. So instead of asking Yuri for a request or a favor in the way I would ask a friend, I was asking with a sense of entitlement and expectation, giving off the vibe that he *should want to do it* because he loves me.

When we talked about it, Yuri realized that many of his expectations of me at home—that I should take care of the house and of him—were a direct result of how his mother had taken care of his family when he was growing up.

This was when I started wondering: what other expectations had we both absorbed from our upbringings that were driving the way we defined and interpreted love, as well as contributing to so many misunderstandings and arguments?

Most of us know that the way we think and behave is largely influenced by our families, but many of us are not conscious of how heavily our family conditioning drives the way we perceive love and relationships.

This is why it's so important to practice asking ourselves *where* our reaction is originating. We have to identify the source of our negative feelings and see if they arise from the various expectations we have that are influenced by our family conditioning.

It also helps to remember that our partners also have preferences and habits shaped by their family conditioning, so when they don't subscribe to something that we believe in, it's not because our partners are opposing us, it's that they genuinely cannot see what we see because their habits and preferences are completely different.

Now that we're aware of this, we can ask ourselves why we get upset when someone behaves differently from what we would expect of them and examine if it's in any way linked to our parents' preferences or even societal influences.

This awareness can enable us to let go of many expectations that we thought were ours, but which could merely be society's or our parents' expectations. Even something as simple as our thoughts on whether a situation is fair or unfair could change significantly.

Sometimes, you might be bothered that your partner doesn't have a lot of money or that your partner is of a different religion, but it's worthwhile to consider that maybe you yourself actually have no issues with it—it may be a concern that you absorbed from other people. Even if you come to the conclusion that it is indeed your personal preference, then you can communicate it as your preference as opposed to communicating it in the form of an expectation. The communication approach would be, "I would like this because..." rather than, "You should be like this."

Family conditioning leads to conscious and subconscious expectations, but now that we're adults with relationships of our own, we need to use our awareness of this conditioning in re-examining our judgements, prejudices, and expectations so that we can decide to let go of those that don't serve us.

THERE ARE NO UNSPOKEN RULES IN THE HUMAN REALM

<Understanding>

I was having a conversation with a friend about expectations in a relationship and the subject of reasonable expectations came up. "Most expectations aren't good for a relationship," he said, "unless they are reasonable ones."

"For example, I would expect my wife to take turns picking up our kid from school, because that's part of the responsibility of being a parent," he explained.

"But if you guys didn't talk about it beforehand, how would she know it's an expectation?" I asked.

"Some things are obvious, like picking up your kid from school is something she should know as a mother."

When first considered, expecting one's partner to voluntarily split the duties when it comes to raising a child is perfectly reasonable. However, one person's definition of responsibility can be very different from that of another, and just because we are in a relationship with someone doesn't mean that our definitions of responsibility and good parenting will automatically merge. The problem here isn't who should do what, or whose definition of responsibility is more accurate—it is the fact that we assume that it's not necessary to talk about some things. It made me wonder: how many thoughts are there in our heads that we don't discuss with our partners? What are all the expectations we have that are not communicated because we think that they are "obvious"?

One of the most dangerous mindsets is the belief that a relationship implies certain unspoken rules. There are no *unspoken rules* in the human realm—even when you love someone, it doesn't mean that you and your partner will suddenly have identical ideas about what is common sense, nor will you both suddenly develop the same perspectives, standards, and beliefs. If something is important to you, then it's important for you to speak about it.

Common sense is not common, because what is common to me is not common to you. We are different people from different backgrounds with different experiences, all of which have shaped us into who we are today. Multiracial or multicultural relationships may outwardly demonstrate how two people are inherently different, but the truth is that we are all inherently different. Even if you and I are from the exact same race and culture, what is common in my household, in my upbringing, and in the depths of my mind is not necessarily what is common in your household, your upbringing, and the depths of your mind.

Just because someone loves us, it doesn't mean that they will automatically know, understand, or even agree with what is in our minds and hearts.

When a partner doesn't do something we believe they should do, we create our own suffering when we immediately equate this with lack of concern on their part and conclude, *"He doesn't care enough, that's why he didn't do it,"* or *"She is irresponsible for not doing that,"* because that is not the absolute truth—it only seems that way from the perspective of *our* reality.

If we insist on holding others to our own standards of what "love" or "responsibility" should look like, then we won't have either the patience or the right mindset to look for the answers as to why our partner are the way they are.

Again, not having expectations does not mean being a pushover or just letting things slide. When our partner's actions have created a serious problem—like failing to pick up his or her child—it warrants an equally serious conversation. However, if we cannot let go of the initial hurt, disappointment, or anger, then the conversation will center around accusation, blame, and guilt instead of actually solving the problem by figuring out *why* it happened and how to change that in the future.

Some people are more considerate than others. Some people are more careless than others. Some people are more selfish than others. It means that we are human, and as such, we are all works

in progress. If we *choose* to be with someone, we cannot hold
them to the same standards that we expect ourselves to uphold,
because we will keep getting upset when they don't meet those
standards. And people will always keep failing if we keep having
expectations of them, because logically, how can someone meet
our standards or expectations when there are actually unspoken
relationship rules?

The exact opposite of taking responsibility for our own happiness
is to expect our partners to know what we need to be happy.
What we need to understand is that while it is absolutely normal
to have needs and desires and preferences, what is not a winning
proposition for our happiness is to expect our partners to know
what those needs, desires, and preferences are, because if we don't
tell them, how would they know?

We need to speak about the things that are important to us, from
the big things such as what you think parenting should be like
to the smallest things; for example, how you feel about having
unwashed dishes in the sink and how often you'd like both of you
to have dinner with your parents, and vice versa.

Many of us feel like we've *already* communicated with our
partner—we've told them these things a million times, and we
may feel we're talking to a brick wall. However, *telling* someone
something isn't communicating—we're just telling them.

When there is even a little bit of resentment in the relationship,
neither party feels safe or secure with the other. This is why
identifying our subconscious expectations is important, because if
you don't even know what it is you expect your partner to give to
you and aren't able to be honest enough with yourself about why
you want it, then you won't be able to explain it to them.

Communication is two-way, so even though we may have very
valid points and reasons for discussion, one of the most important
aspects of communication is to allow the other person to express
their opinions and beliefs without getting offended or upset.

When we are coming from this mindset and perspective, we will
seek to explain our needs instead of holding on to expectations
that only hurt us and the relationship. We will seek to understand

our partner better instead of feeling upset at not being understood. Then, it becomes easier to let go of all the hurt and anger and remove the layers of indignation, self-righteousness, and defensiveness that make communication difficult.

EVEN IF WHAT IS IMPORTANT TO YOU ISN'T IMPORTANT TO YOUR PARTNER, IT DOES NOT MEAN THAT *YOU* ARE UNIMPORTANT

<Understanding>

A few years ago, my friend Mikayla met a guy and they started dating. They would hang out at her house on the weekends. My friend had recycling bins in her house where she would separate her trash. The first few times her boyfriend came over, he would throw everything into one bin. Aghast, she told him, "Different materials go into different bins!" and she would reach into the bin to dig around in the trash to remove what he'd put in.

In response, he said, "Why do you bother recycling?"

In all fairness, recycling was not a common practice in Malaysia, and most people are not in the habit of doing it with their items for disposal.

"How do you know the garbage collectors won't just grab all the bags and just throw them into the truck anyway?" he asked. "They won't separate the trash, and it'll be a waste of your efforts."

"Well, I don't know if they will or they won't, but it's something *I* want to do," she explained.

"Hah, good luck with that!" he replied.

So, in light of his deep belief that it would be pointless to recycle, she told him that he didn't have to do it. She did, however, requested that he not throw anything into the bins when he came over and instead leave the trash on the counter so that she could sort them out later.

He agreed, and that was the end of that conversation. They spent the rest of the day in her apartment rather peacefully.

"Weren't you upset?" I asked when she told me what had happened.

"A little, yes," she said.

"So how did you let it go so easily and not argue about it?" I asked; "It must have affected your level of respect for him." Recycling is one of the fundamental beliefs in her life, and I can imagine that it must be important to her that her partner also recycles.

She said to me, "Well, I was thinking to myself that if I wanted him to *do* what I do, it would already be one battle; and if I wanted him to *believe* what I believe, it would be two battles."

"Besides, I wouldn't want anyone imposing their beliefs on me, so I wouldn't want to do that to him," she pointed out.

This sounded extremely logical. My friend understood that recycling—however important to her—was *her* belief.

The reason she didn't take offense at his comments or became angry was because she understood that he wasn't disagreeing because he didn't love her or wasn't supportive of her—he disagreed because he was genuinely voicing his opinion as to what *he* believed to be true.

Most of the time, when someone disagrees with us, we think that they are *objecting* to us, especially if they are disagreeing about something that is one of our fundamental beliefs.

However, that's not true—people are not objecting to *us*, they are telling us what *they* believe. If we can see it from this point of view, then it's so much easier to listen to our partner's differing opinions without perceiving them as attacks or objections. Again, no matter how personal it feels, we have to learn not to take it personally.

It also helps to understand that even when we've conveyed to our partner what is important to us, it may not be important to them—not because *we* are not important to them, but *the thing* is not something that they agree with or even necessarily understand.

If we immediately equate someone's unwillingness to subscribe to
what we believe in or give us what we need as *"It means you don't
care enough!"* then we will suffer. And why would you want to
suffer when it is *not* the truth?

The truth is that a person *can* love and care deeply about us yet
have differing beliefs and values, because they are an entirely
different human being. It doesn't make sense for us to be unhappy
when our partner is not receptive to us imposing our beliefs
on them.

IT'S NOT PERSONAL, EVEN WHEN IT FEELS PERSONAL

<Understanding>

In the early stages of my relationship with Yuri, we had a huge argument about the death penalty.

I remember it vividly because we were having the conversation in the car, and we couldn't get out of the car even though we'd reached our destination because we hadn't yet finished talking (that is, arguing).

We were just having a casual conversation about capital punishment until Yuri mentioned that he doesn't believe in the death penalty. I was taken aback and asked him, "But what about people who commit murder? Don't you think they deserve it?"

Yuri believes there is no evil, only ignorance. He told me, "There are many reasons why people commit murder, and there is a chance they can be rehabilitated. To kill someone because they murder someone else is to say that there is no chance for rehabilitation, but that's more convenience than truth. Taking a life for another life is the same ignorant act perpetuating itself."

Looking back, I don't think I was even properly listening. When he was talking, all I was thinking was, *I don't agree.*

"What if *I* was killed? Or your *mother*? Would you still think that?" I asked incredulously.

I was so upset that I surprised even myself. I wasn't even aware that I had such a strong opinion on this issue, yet I was so affected by Yuri's opposing belief. I remember being really angry with him even though he hadn't actually *done* anything to me.

It was only later that I came to understand myself better. When I examined *why* I had reacted so personally to something that wasn't even personal, I realized that I associated his stance against capital punishment with an unwillingness to fight for the people he loved. It felt a lot like he cared more about his belief than he did about me. And if I was to be very honest, I hated how his views were on a higher moral ground than mine, which highlighted that perhaps I wasn't a very "good" person for believing in the death penalty in the first place.

When I came to these realizations about my own behavior, I could see how his belief was not a reflection of how little he cared about the lives of the people he loved. I just had to ask myself, "Do you *really* believe that he wouldn't care if you were murdered?" And the answer was a resounding *no*. I believe that he does care and would feel the pain deeply. It was like a switch went off in my head—I believe that he loves me, and I can clearly see that his beliefs have nothing to do with me; they are part of who he is. It reminded me of the fact that even when someone loves us, they are still their own person.

As it turns out, Yuri taught me something incredibly valuable. When I stopped being upset, I could actually think about my own views toward justice and revenge. I used to think that loyalty was demonstrated in a very specific way, and that love is reflected in your loved ones' desire to hurt the people who hurt you.

It wasn't until he offered me another viewpoint that I began to consider for myself whether my definitions of love and loyalty were healthy or logical. When I examined that, I realized that "an eye for an eye" just makes the world more blind. Justice is a man-made concept, where the only thing we may get is satisfaction but it does nothing to help the pain or hate. The lessons I learned in this process resulted in my writing and making many videos on my thoughts on forgiveness and letting go.

You could say that I agreed with Yuri in the end, but it wasn't a battle about whose belief was better. What inspired me was that *he* didn't need me to think like him. He didn't judge me or have less respect for me when I told him I believed in capital punishment. He simply offered his own belief as a point of discussion, which turned into an argument because I took it very personally, which then set off a chain reaction of us being angry with each other.

When we are upset with people, it is the perfect opportunity to learn more about ourselves. When you don't agree with someone, it's not that the other person is always wrong, it's that they have a different belief. It's not that you are wrong, either, it's that you have a different belief.

And when we give ourselves the chance to ponder someone else's differing point of view, we might discover new perspectives that enhance our lives in terms of growth and maturity.

WHEN SOMEONE WE LOVE GIVES US WHAT WE NEED, IT IS A GIFT, NOT OUR ENTITLEMENT

<Perspective>

It would be nice not to have needs, because I would imagine we'd have complete contentment...a place where it's not that we don't need people, but that we don't need anything from external sources to be happy with our identities and our lives.

However, for those of us who still have needs, it's not a bad thing at all—learning about ourselves is the big adventure of being human, and our ability to identify and understand our own needs has a direct impact on whether our lives are happy or painful adventures.

When we fall in love, we naturally bring our needs into the relationship, consciously or subconsciously. Taking responsibility for our happiness means taking responsibility for what we want and what we need—it's the acknowledgment of *"I* have a need" instead of thinking, *"You* are *supposed* to do that because you said you love me."

There is a fine yet very distinct difference between the two.

The first is where we understand that when someone is able to give to us something in the way we need, it is a *gift* and a privilege. When our partner subscribes to our views and beliefs and does what we want, it is appreciated and very much valued.

The latter is where we expect our special someone to give us what we want because of love. When our partners don't subscribe to our views or beliefs, we get upset and end up feeling unhappy. When they do give us what we want, we're happy, but it doesn't feel like a bonus, because when we believe that doing so is our partners' duty, it's the "right" and "normal" thing to do anyway.

Most of the time, it's not our partners doing something "wrong" that makes us unhappy. It is usually because they have good intentions but don't know what our norms or deep-rooted needs are, so they have no idea what will trigger our sensitivities and defensiveness. They likely don't know that we feel attacked, unsupported, or rejected; all they know is that we are upset.

For them to understand us, we have to first understand ourselves. This is one of the main reasons why expectations work against us—our minds are too busy focusing on thinking, "*You should know, you should care!*" to even go down the other avenue of, "*Why is this so important to me, and how do I put into words what I am feeling?*"

Our minds can only focus on one direction at a time. When we don't let go of our expectations, the concept of "should" paves the way for our emotions to overtake us. Our communication tools will then consist of conveying our hurt, disappointment, desperation, and anger.

However, when we let go of expectations, our minds can go down the other direction of trying to understand ourselves and our needs better so we can find the right words to express why something is so important to us. Our communication tools will consist of conveying why *we would feel* rejected, attacked, unsupported, disregarded, disrespected, insignificant, worthless, and so on. In this direction of thinking, we are able to take it less personally.

For example, we can understand that our partner is not *purposefully* trying to disrespect us, it's just that the manner in which they think and behave leads to us *feeling* disrespected. This helps us to look inward to examine what our sensitivities, fears, needs, and desires are, so that we can better understand why we are so easily triggered by certain behavior.

When we love someone, we tell them "*I love you;*" we don't say, "*I love you because you make me feel....*"

However, the majority of us are in relationships because our partners are giving us something we need. If we acknowledge this, we remind ourselves that when we choose to love someone, we are saying we *love that person*, full stop. When we convey our needs to our partner, it is a request, not a demand; which means that if they are able to give us what we need, it is a gift, not an obligation. Nothing is owed to us, because it is our choice to love.

The way we communicate in a relationship changes drastically when we are honest about what we need instead of mistakenly thinking that our partner *should* give it to us if they love us.

This does not mean that we need to abolish all our needs before we can have a happy relationship, but it does mean that when we take responsibility for our own needs, we are able to identify *why* we are unhappy.

OUR ABILITY TO LOVE IS ONLY AS GOOD AS OUR SKILLS

<Understanding>

When my dad had an affair and left my mom to be with someone else, it was an act of betrayal of the vows he made to my mom when they got married. My mom and our family did feel betrayed, but at the same time, we understood how it could have happened.

My dad took on the roles of a husband and a father, but he is also a human being with his own beliefs, needs, and fears. He didn't suddenly gain any superpowers just because he got married and had children. All his insecurities and fears did not disappear. If anything, they were amplified over time because he wasn't consciously working on them.

A person can love another human being, but their capacity to love is tied to their mental strength, emotional maturity, and self-development skills, and none of these automatically grow unless we work on them.

My dad's actions weren't responsible as a husband or a father; but as human beings, our ability to execute our responsibilities requires more than just good intentions or even genuine desire—we need to develop the skills. It is similar to how being promoted to a position as a manager doesn't automatically make you a good leader. You need to develop and hone your managerial skills to have the ability to be an effective and inspiring leader.

Likewise, the desire of each of us to be a great person is different from our ability to be self-aware and giving. We feel like we're trying really hard and yet in reality don't see consistent results. It is like having good intentions to lose weight while lacking the discipline and the technique to actually do it. My dad was unhappy in the family not because he didn't try—he tried his best, but his best was only as good as his skills.

When we try very hard to communicate with our partners, we often expect them to be able to *understand* us and *agree* with us, as well as to have the *capabilities* to act upon it. However, we can only *convey* our beliefs, desires, and needs to our partners. That's the best we can do. We forget that it's already hard enough for someone to understand a concept likely to be foreign to them (because to us, it feels like common sense). We forget that even when one's partner does understand, it's only logical that they might not agree because they are a different human being. We also forget that even if they *do understand and agree*, they might not have the *ability* to give us what we want.

This is why we are always so frustrated after having the same argument over and over again. It's almost natural to come to the conclusion that our partner doesn't care enough, because otherwise *why* are they still doing what they know hurts us or isn't healthy for the relationship?

It is our expectations and projections of what love should be that create our suffering. For example, we could be good friends with someone who isn't great at talking about his or her feelings, and we wouldn't be upset. But if the next day our friendship status turned into a romantic relationship, we're likely to get really upset when the person doesn't tell us what they're thinking. But the thing is, the person *has not changed*—they are still the same person with the same habits and the same uncommunicative personality— it is our *expectations* of the person that have changed.

In a way, love blinds us to how challenging relationships can be. Love is such a wondrous feeling that it makes us feel like we can *intuitively* overcome insurmountable challenges, but we have to be mindful that love only serves to motivate us to want to try. And this is the thing—*wanting* to try doesn't always mean we *have the abilities* and capabilities needed to do so—this is why loving someone doesn't automatically mean that we know how to love, especially in the way that our beloved wants to be loved.

This is why it's so important for us to examine *why* we choose to be in a relationship with someone in the first place. If we insist on being loved in a very specific way and our partner has neither the skills nor the ability to give it to us, then choosing to stay in the relationship means we *accept* them for who they are. Because otherwise, we will keep saying we love someone yet feel constantly irritated, hurt, and angry with them, which is how we cause our own suffering.

Sometimes we can think, *"He has the ability! He just chooses not to give me what I need!"* But that's like saying, *"You have two arms and two legs, why can't you work out every day and eat healthy and lose weight?"* A person's ability to do something depends on more than just their physical and mental capacities, it's also their ability to be internally instead of externally motivated—the ability to understand their own ego, needs, and fears as well as the ability to take responsibility for their own happiness.

This is why in a relationship, the feeling of love is not enough. Someone can truly love us, but they don't level up in their ability just because they love us. Some people are messier than others, or more forgetful than others, or more selfish than others, and even when they *try very hard* to not be that way, we might think they're not trying hard enough because we are comparing their results to what *we* would do.

Similarly, we can truly love our partner, but we don't develop magical skills no matter how strong our love is. This is why we can love someone desperately, yet feel desperately unhappy; because no human being is able to fully love and fully give in a relationship unless we also learn how to develop a healthy relationship with ourselves.

EVERYONE HAS THEIR OWN JOURNEY, AND NOBODY IS OBLIGATED TO US

<Perspective>

As human beings, we have roles to play and responsibilities to fulfill, be it in our relationships or in our careers. However, no matter what roles we take on, it is important to remember that we are all still individual human beings, and every one of us has a journey that we need to take during our time here on earth.

In order to come to realize the crucial lessons we need to learn in this lifetime, we sometimes have to take other roads, even if it's a more painful or difficult journey. It is similar to how we won't heed people's advice about avoiding a dangerous hole in the ground—we need to walk straight in and fall before coming to the realization of what it means to be mindful. Some lessons are only learned through experiences of discomfort. Most of the time, what we learn in life isn't what anybody can teach us—it is our own enlightenment as to what it means to be happy through the journey we are taking that is our core learning.

As far as my parents' divorce, am I disappointed that my dad made the choices he did? Very much so. But do I hold it against him? No.

Even though my dad had a role and responsibilities as a father, there are lessons in gratitude, love, and patience that my dad really needed to learn as a human being—he needed to understand how happiness cannot be found externally, because it exists within us— and unfortunately, he couldn't learn these lessons while he was with our family.

We all make our choices, and whichever path we choose to take will shape the life we will live. Regardless of what roles we all play, when two people cross paths in life, it is always a privilege, not an obligation. Everyone has a choice in life. People don't have to take care of us. They don't have to cook for us or pay for us. They don't have to take care of us when we're old. They don't have to love us. When they do, it's a *choice* they make over and over again, and we can never take that choice for granted. We can be in the role of a husband, wife, father, mother, brother, sister or child, but nobody can force us into a loving relationship with someone just because it "should be that way." This is why when someone gives us love, it is always such an amazing gift, and it is not to be viewed as their obligation to do so.

When we understand that it is a privilege to be involved in the lives of the people we love—as opposed to thinking that people owe us something just because they made a promise or took on a role—we can truly appreciate our family even more.

This was such an important realization for me, especially in the early years of my marriage. I realized that even though my husband had signed a paper and promised to love and cherish me, his love and acts of love are always a gift and a privilege. When we look at our relationships this way, it is so much easier to be grateful for the people in our lives.

PEOPLE CAN LOVE US, BUT THEY CANNOT COMPLETE US

<Self-Love>

When we start dating, it is not surprising that it's instinctive for us to look toward our partners to complete us and give us fulfilment. We seek love for its promise to lighten up our dark days, for its strength to support our weaknesses, and for its ability to heal what is broken inside.

Too often, however, we associate *need* with *love*. When someone needs us, it makes us feel important and significant, so it's also natural to assume that needing someone is a sign of our love for them. This is why concepts like *"You complete me"* and *"I would sacrifice anything for you"* become a subconscious benchmark for what true love is—we aspire to be all that someone needs, and we are prepared to sacrifice for our partner and expect the same in return.

The problem with this is that nobody can really complete us. It's not that love is a farce and movies lie, it's just that no matter how much someone love us, they can only *support* us through our own journey of self-love, self-healing, and self-acceptance. They cannot *give* fulfilment to us, no matter how hard they try.

When we need someone to give to us in a very specific manner, it's because there are needs that we need to fill; and these needs create gaps inside us that heavily influence our definition of what love is.

This is why some of us have a hard time leaving toxic relationships—we recognize the toxicity, but because the person fills a very important gap we have within us, other problems—even abuse—can be endured because there's a fear of losing someone who can fulfil those needs in our life.

Sometimes we're not even aware that we have gaps that we need people to fill, but if we keep seeing patterns of how our relationships play out, it is an indication that we need to look inward. If we have fears of abandonment, we'll be happy as long as the person gives us a sense of security and a measure of comfort. If we fear that we aren't good enough, we'll be happy when our partner validates us. As long as our partner continuously fills up that gap within us, we will feel like we're in equilibrium—like we're happy. However, people are always changing, and when they do, the balance will suddenly change too—either the gaps we need to fill get better or the person simply stops filling those gaps.

This was what happened to my parents' relationship. My father loved my mother—more than he himself knew, I suspect—but he had massive gaps in his life that he needed to fill to be happy. For many years, my mom was filling those gaps of self-doubt and insecurity for him. With her, he felt whole, secure, and confident. However, over the years, those gaps widened and changed, and he needed more and more validation in life.

Sometimes, the reason we are still unhappy even when our partners are giving us what we need is because they might not be giving it in the *measure* that we need, and that's the problem. When we don't know how to give to ourselves what we seek, the gaps become so wide that it can be hard for anyone to give us everything we need to fill them. Even when someone is giving us a lot emotionally, they might not always be able to fill those gaps equally and perfectly, and that's a big part of the reason why we might feel that our partner is not giving enough or not being supportive enough.

This is why love often isn't enough in a relationship, because no matter how much we love someone, we can carry with us unresolved emotional insecurities, fears of conflict and abandonment, and a deep need for validation that makes it incredibly difficult for us to be happy in our relationships. Only we can remove what blocks our happiness, peeling away the layers one by one like an onion; and that often means recognizing what the gaps are in our lives and working on filling them ourselves. To do that, we need to put aside our egos in order to shed the layers of blame and resentment and be able to reflect internally. This requires an honesty where we are willing to feel extremely *uncomfortable.*

To be happy in love is to examine what our fears and insecurities are. Do we fear conflict, insignificance, and rejection? What is it that we tend to seek from others? What do we need in order to feel significant and worthy? When we examine it deeply, we might find that the source of our expectations isn't coming from what is "normal" or "fair" for a loving partner to give, but rather from what we *need* a partner to give in order for us to feel complete.

To be happy in love, the journey begins with identifying what we need so that we can work on the little ways in which we can give happiness to ourselves, instead of seeking it externally with each relationship. We cannot escape the work we have to do for ourselves.

We study so that we can have a successful career, but one of the most important lessons in life is learning how to value ourselves so we don't look to another human being to give us a sense of worthiness. You are only enough if *you* believe it, not if someone else believes it. We can only take responsibility for our own happiness when we don't rely on someone else to complete us.

WE DON'T FIND FULFILMENT IN OTHER PEOPLE; WE FIND FULFILMENT BY LOOKING INWARDS

<Self-Love>

Love of the romantic variety frequently comes easy; we don't have to *try* to fall in love. The feeling of love is very similar to the feeling of happiness, where the emotion floods our senses and it feels more euphoric than words can describe. A *relationship*, however, is very different from love, because a relationship requires more than just emotion, no matter how strong the emotion is.

The nature of human beings is that if we cannot fulfil ourselves, we will be unfulfilled no matter where we go, what we do, or who our companions are. We cannot "find ourselves" by going away and escaping. This is why we can take vacations and be immersed in distractions yet feel equally depressed afterward when we are back home and alone—because we're back at square one (and probably also more depressed because now we're a lot more broke).

We "find ourselves" by digging deep within. We do it from stillness and the willingness to go through the pain of being honest about who we are and what we need. The biggest challenge in life isn't what life throws at us, but how willing we are to look into the mirror without denial and clearly see all our fears, insecurities, and what we don't like about ourselves.

It is natural for us to start wondering if someone is right for us when we are not happy in a relationship, but to determine that, we have to first question what lies within us before we start to look outside at other people.

Before we delve into how to be happy in a relationship, we need to examine how we can be happy with ourselves. Before we can have a healthy relationship with someone else, we need to have a healthy relationship with ourselves. Before we know how to love someone else, we need to learn how to love ourselves.

Loving ourselves is not about thinking that we are perfect but about that willingness to look within, let go of the desire to take shelter in denial, and really see all our fears, inadequacies, and the things we don't like about ourselves. Because it is only when we are honest with ourselves about our own needs and desires that we do not subconsciously seek validation, attention, and significance from those to whom we are attracted. Otherwise, we will find ourselves experiencing the pattern of having one unhappy relationship after another.

This doesn't mean that we have to be perfect before we can be in a relationship, it just means that we have to learn how to give love and respect to ourselves before we can be *happy* in one. Fulfilment only comes when we start learning how to fill our own need and gaps, because the more we need external validation, the more we tend to self-destruct while seeking it. If we don't learn how to nourish ourselves, to give ourselves what we need and what we seek, we will only be able to be temporarily satisfied with our lives and never truly content.

This is so important, because when we don't know how to love ourselves, it makes it difficult for us to have a happy relationship with someone, a relationship where we are there because we *want* to have a life with this person rather than because we feel like we cannot live without them.

"BUT IT'S ONLY FAIR!" IS A CONCEPT THAT BRINGS A GREAT DEAL OF MISERY

<Awareness>

One of the questions I get asked the most often is, *"But isn't it fair to expect one's partner to also give back?"*

What expectations are fair is a subject that many of us feel strongly about, which is why suffering and misery are such constants in our relationships.

When it comes to our romantic relationships, most of us commit to a relationship without talking about the nitty-gritty of our personal preferences and expectations. We depend on the emotion of love to carry us through, and then we try to figure things out along the way.

Figuring out things along the way is typical in most relationships. With our partner, as we get to know each other better, we discover things that we never would have known before we got together. In this process of being together and starting to understand each other, there will be moments when we're surprised, shocked, taken aback, hurt, disappointed, and angry. These feelings are brought on by the fact that we trust this person, and we are also at our most vulnerable because we have opened our hearts to them.

However, there's nothing wrong with this. If you think about it, all the emotions we experience in relationships are a completely normal part of how two human beings learn to understand each other and work out ways to live and love together. At this point, what is crucial for us to know is this: although figuring out the relationship is a necessary process, the concept of fairness *isn't* a necessary part of the process.

Being upset with each other is natural, but what makes it a problem is when we don't know how to work things out without accusation, blame, and resentment. When two different people come together, it's not negative at all to find that there are differing opinions and beliefs. What *is* negative is the concept of fair expectations.

When we go into a relationship with someone, it is similar to willingly entering a contract. We may not have signed an agreement on paper, but the fact that we *want* to be in the relationship means we have agreed to it. However, if we were to broker a deal and sign a contract, we would first negotiate until we were satisfied with the terms. But we don't do that when it comes to our relationships—when we love someone, we usually dive headlong into a relationship. So we basically have agreed to a contract where we are *happy* not knowing the terms, so how can we say it's unfair when we find out later that the terms are not very satisfactory and bring unexpected problems?

It is only natural to find out *later* that our partner has preferences, values, habits, or beliefs that are different from ours; but of course, it can still take us completely by surprise. You might find that your partner does do things you would not do or does not communicate the way you communicate, and they may very well not show you love the way you show them love.

The thing is, even if we think that the terms greatly favor the other party, *we* willingly signed the contract. In other words, we chose to enter the relationship of our own free will. And here's the important part—we are willingly *choosing to stay* in the relationship, even if we think the terms are not favorable. So if we *choose it,* how can we think that it's unfair when we don't get what we want or need?

We know we can exit a relationship when we feel miserable, yet often we love our partners and can't bring ourselves to leave. However, we're not happy—we have resentment for the person because we feel like we're being shortchanged or unappreciated, and we feel that it's not fair. We can leave, but we want to stay. But we feel it's unfair. Can you see how it is *this dilemma*—and not our partner—that is the cause of all our frustration?

Most of us, going by instinct, will withdraw or hold back if we sense that the other person isn't going to give as well. When we make an effort with the belief that it should be *fair*, what happens is that we will try for a little bit and then withdraw when we don't get the response we want. Then, after some time has passed, we'll try to make an effort again, only to give up and be even more upset when we don't get the response we want. We will repeat the same pattern over and over again, feeling more and more frustrated in the process. In the end, we'll surmise that it must be the other person's fault—because we have genuinely tried. In reality, the problem isn't about whose fault it is, the problem is that the concept of fairness is perpetuating anger, righteousness, and judgement, all of which make it so difficult for us to communicate without arguing.

In order to communicate and work through relationship problems, we need to practice loving kindness and understanding; not because we *should*, but because that is the *best* and most workable way to keep a conversation open, honest, and safe. For us to bring down walls and make a conversation more open and less emotionally charged, we have to first drop the concept of fair expectations.

WHEN WE GIVE (WITHOUT EXPECTATIONS), WE RECEIVE

<Understanding>

In our marriage, Yuri used to *want* me to contribute equally to doing the household chores, which he felt was fair. Whether or not it was fair, it made me feel like I was constantly being measured for how good of a wife I was, and not only did that made me feel guilty, it also made me feel defensive.

At the time, I was hosting and producing a breakfast show on radio, which meant getting up at four o'clock every morning. I was constantly tired from the lack of sleep, and I felt my husband wasn't being supportive or had little empathy for what I was going through. I also had expectations of what love and marriage ought to be, and I had thoughts like, "*If you loved me, you would understand this, or do that*" running through my head, which added suffering to my state of mind.

We tried so hard to communicate what we needed from each other, yet we each felt like the other person just couldn't understand nor give what was needed. Our conversations would be fraught with frustration, impatience, anger, and most of all, hurt. We would both be incredibly defensive as well as offensive during these interactions. This drove us further and further apart until one day...I realized that something had changed.

The *vibe* in the house had changed; it had become more positive. I wish I could take the credit for it, but it was a conscious effort on Yuri's part. I noticed that Yuri had been doing the house chores without the usual need for me to *also* contribute. He was doing the chores *happily*, which was a vibe that was absent before. It was so strange—he didn't say anything, but because he wasn't displaying his usual moodiness or reluctance about doing the house chores, I could *feel* that he had dropped his expectations of what was "fair" and what I "should contribute" in the relationship.

He seemed happy and was loving even when *I* hadn't actually done or changed anything, which led me to feel like he wasn't judging me anymore and that he didn't resent me for not contributing. Even though he didn't do anything romantic or undertake any grand gestures, I started to feel more loved.

When I asked him about this months later, Yuri told me that the changes in him started when he decided to be happy. He said that he went through a process of asking himself if he wanted to grow old with me. His answer was *yes*, so he decided that since he valued the relationship, *something* had to change. He was thinking, "How can I shift my perspective in a way that can make me happier?"

He figured that he had nothing to lose and everything to gain. He felt that if he was happy, the relationship might be happier. And even if the relationship didn't improve, he would be a happier person, and for him, that was already a win.

To be happy, he decided that he was just going to do what he thought should be done. If he wanted the clothes washed more often, he would happily do it without expecting me to also contribute. If the dirty dishes in the sink bothered him, he would wash them instead of telling me to do it. Previously, he used to wonder, "What is the point of a marriage if I have to do all the chores on my own?" To be happier, he shifted his perspective to, "If I lived alone, I would have no problem doing the chores anyway."

This might seem self-sacrificial, like he had the losing end of the stick, but he didn't view it that way, because he wasn't doing it for me, he was doing it for *himself*—he wanted this relationship, and he wanted to be happy.

With that small shift of perspective, so much change happened. He met both of his goals. He was able to drop his notion of fairness and equality in the relationship—resulting in him feeling less frustrated and less resentful—and he was so much happier, because the clothes were always nicely laundered and the sink always clear of dishes!

Yuri started practicing this state of mind long before I took notice, and in those long weeks and months, he didn't resent the fact that I did not notice or give anything back. He had no expectations of me giving back what he contributed, yet he didn't feel he was being a pushover or that he was being taken advantage of in the situation. This was only possible because he reminded himself that he was *choosing* to be with me. He also reminded himself that he didn't have to *outsource his happiness* to me just because I was his wife. This clarity and his resultant decision gave him enough motivation to try his best to fulfil his own needs instead of relying or depending on my actions to give him happiness.

When it comes to love and relationships, who should give first or who should give more is not dependent upon what is fairer. Fairness doesn't even play a part in it, because in reality, it is the person who is *more capable* of giving—the person who has more wisdom, more maturity, and more motivation—who will be the one to give.

People might perceive a person who gives more as weak, but in truth, it is because they are so much stronger and more capable that they are able to see the wisdom and gain insight on how to be happy and how to love someone. Only a person who values themselves highly will start to take positive actions for their own happiness instead of needing another to give it to them.

My respect, admiration, and awe for Yuri grew so much after this sequence of events. He made himself happy, and in the process, inspired me to also do the same. We started to be able to talk more without arguing, because the resentment that was permeating our relationship was slowly ebbing away. I felt like he didn't need me to "be this" or "be that" in order to love me. I felt accepted for who I was, and as a result, no longer felt a need to be so defensive.

If Yuri had *waited* for me to give first, or if he had tried and then given up when he didn't see me responding, none of the positive changes in our relationship would have happened. Our frustrations about each other would have caused so much resentment that it would have eaten our relationship alive. He started the ball rolling, and it really helped me.

It usually isn't one person's fault when there are problems in a relationship, so the natural inclination is that when we make an effort, we also want the *other person* to make an effort. It's only fair. And again, the concept of fair expectations holds us back—we will likely be very resentful if the other person isn't making the kind of effort we are making. Every time we try, we feel like we are sacrificing if our partner doesn't reciprocate. For every effort we put in, we feel even more angry when the person doesn't seem to appreciate it.

Sooner or later, it becomes a stalemate—nobody wants to give an inch unless the other also gives. No one makes enough of an effort, and the relationship deteriorates. This is what happens if we insist on staying in a relationship as well as insist that things change, because no matter how hard we try, we cannot force another person to change. There is only one variable, and the variable is not the *other* person.

Yuri wanted change, and so he changed himself instead of expecting me to change.

When you remove expectations, you remove resentment. When you remove resentment, you'd be surprised at how you can listen better when you communicate. There's less judgement and more patience; fewer hurtful things said and more kindness given. The most interesting thing of all is that when you remove expectations from the equation, people feel more compelled to give.

The irony is this: We have expectations because we want something from someone. But in order to get what we want, we have to not expect it in the first place. We cannot pretend to have no expectations, because no matter how nice or patient we make an effort to be about it, people can always feel the weight of our expectations upon them. But when we drop our expectations, we are able to make the necessary effort without feeling like it's so unfair that they're not making a similar effort back.

What can really help is to be really clear about what we want in the first place. What is your true objective? Yuri wanted things to be fair, but that wasn't actually his objective. His objectives were to have a happy relationship and for himself to be happy. So when he focused on his *true* objectives, it became so much easier to give without expectations, because he knew *why* he was giving—and it was not to get a reaction or response.

When we give without expectations, we start to receive. That is the law of the universe. When people are free to make their own choices, when they don't feel measured or judged, when they feel accepted and safe...they start to give.

Even if they don't, you'll have learned the valuable skills necessary to making yourself happy. Either way, you win.

DON'T OUTSOURCE
YOUR HAPPINESS TO
YOUR PARTNER

<Awareness>

When Yuri and I got married, I was twenty-seven years old, he was four years older, and we both definitely expected the other person to make us happy. It wasn't a conscious thought—we weren't thinking, "*Oh, you want to marry me? That means you have to make me happy!*" In fact, it was such a subtle expectation that we didn't even know that we believed in it.

We were both aware that our happiness is always our choice. However, we felt like *marriage* is different—both of us subconsciously thought that when you take on vows to care for someone and when you make a commitment toward a relationship, it means that you are also taking on responsibility for your partner's happiness. It wasn't until a few difficult years later that we started to question the wisdom of that. Is it actually true that love is about making each other happy?

There were times when neither of us enjoyed being with each other very much because we would often fight, yet we weren't unhappy enough to leave the relationship, either. The thing is, we had really enjoyed each other's company when we were just friends. So what had changed?

When I examined the way we interacted with each other, I realized that very little had changed about our interaction. It was the way we *responded* to each other that had changed. When we were friends, we weren't as sensitive or defensive. We didn't have any requirements or conditions or expectations of each other. But the moment we started dating, it was like we were seeing the same person through a different lens. We each saw the each other differently, but in reality, we were still the *exact same people.*

The reason I tried so hard to understand the difference between a friendship and a couple relationship is because I wanted to know *why* I was so bothered by things I didn't used to be bothered about before. And that was when I came to the realization that I had given a great deal of the responsibility for my own happiness over to Yuri—if he did this, it made me happy; if he didn't do that, it made me unhappy.

The most illogical thing was that I thought I *deserved* to hold him accountable for my unhappiness, because I thought that's what love was. You're supposed to make each other happy! Yuri felt the same, and so what ended up happening was that we both outsourced our happiness to each other.

All of these feelings were so unconscious that it took a long time for us to realize this. After a lot of heartache and misery, we slowly learned one of the most crucial lessons in love and happiness, and that is: *even when someone loves you, it is not their job to make you happy.*

When people love us, it doesn't mean that they are expected to make us happy, because when we outsource our happiness to someone—when we make our happiness someone else's job, then we'll constantly feel happy or unhappy based on what they do or don't do.

In general, I was pretty good at understanding how to take responsibility for my own happiness. This was why I didn't tend to be affected by how people behaved or get upset when things didn't go as planned. However, it wasn't until a few years into my marriage that I realized what it meant to take responsibility for my own happiness in the *context of a relationship.*

It's ironic how love can blind us to what we can usually see easily. In the context of our lives, so many of us easily understand that we are responsible for our own happiness. However, once we get into a relationship, we find ourselves operating from a different set of rules when it comes to our happiness.

It's so important to understand that even when someone makes a vow to love and cherish us, there *isn't* an implicit vow to take on responsibility for our happiness. People can certainly bring joy into our lives, but nobody can *make* us happy.

Our happiness has always been and will always be our own responsibility. It sounds incredibly strange, but there is an incredible sense of freedom and empowerment that comes with such a realization. When you drop your expectations of how your partner should make you happy, you are free to discover and unearth all the ways *you* can make *yourself* happy.

LOVE IS NOT ABOUT SACRIFICES, BUT ABOUT ACCEPTANCE

<Acceptance>

If our happiness is our own responsibility, what then is love? Why even be in a relationship if we always have to make ourselves happy?

These are very good questions, and questions that we need to answer for ourselves.

Why, indeed? What's in it for us?

Growing up, we think we know what love is. In books, movies, and stories, love is often portrayed through the most romantic sacrifices possible—love is how someone makes you feel and what the person is willing to do for you.

This is why we often willingly and happily sacrifice for our partner, and then when they don't seem willing to make equal amounts, or even a tiny bit of sacrifice, we feel hurt, unloved, and ultimately, resentful.

But perhaps love isn't what someone is willing to do for us or sacrifice for us. Perhaps the truest evidence of love is when someone is willing to accept the responsibility of making *themselves* happy. Because that is the only time when someone is in a relationship with us not for what we can give them, but simply for the fact that they *want* to be there.

Falling in love is easy, but actually loving someone isn't so simple. We can be very good at *doing* things for someone, and we can very good at *sacrificing* for them. But are we able to *accept them for who they are*?

It's not that we love someone and therefore we accept them.

It's not that we accept someone and therefore we love them.

Acceptance *is* love.

This is the biggest challenge in any relationship—to completely accept a partner for who they are. It's incredibly difficult to just accept someone without feeling the need for them to adopt our way of thinking and doing things, our beliefs and values, as well as giving us what we need.

This was what held Yuri and I back. We couldn't accept one another completely—we wanted to tweak a little bit of this and change a little bit of that. So, even as we had so much love for one another, we did not really know what it meant to love someone.

Love is meant to bring two people closer, but lack of acceptance drives people further apart. You can get along swimmingly well, you can have so much in common, and you can love each other's families, but as long as you have expectations that the other person has to change, the love will feel very conditional.

Conditional love makes us afraid. It makes us distrust. It makes us feel like we're being measured all the time. It makes us feel judged. It makes us resentful.

We can be the nicest and sweetest people in the world, we can be attractive and cheerful, we can have integrity and a good heart, but if we do not see how our expectations are sabotaging our relationships, we will always have difficulties truly loving someone.

For most human beings, when we do not feel accepted for who we are, we do not feel safe to be vulnerable with our partners; so we start instinctively protecting ourselves by holding back, and that makes it practically impossible to communicate positively, kindly, or lovingly. All this slowly eats away at the joy of being with the person.

Most of us know how we want to *be* loved, but we will not fully know how to love another human being until we know how to accept people for who they are. The practice of acceptance begins with the willingness to take responsibility for our own happiness, so that we're not blaming our partners when we are not happy.

Why is it that we understand how nobody is perfect, yet when a partner shows us their imperfections, we get so easily upset?

Accepting our partners does not mean that we think they are perfect. It means we see them for who they are, with all their flaws and weaknesses, and we don't judge them for it. It means that we can figure out solutions to problems in the relationship without blame. It means that we can communicate with kindness without being hurtful *even when* we are upset.

It is all this—and not sacrifice—that is love.

EXPECTING SOMEONE TO HAVE NO EXPECTATIONS IS AN EXPECTATION IN ITSELF

<Awareness>

Sometimes, we think that we have no expectations and it is our partners who have very high expectations. But expecting someone to have no expectations is an expectation in itself. It sounds mind-boggling, but when you think about it, it makes sense.

If we think, *"I accept you for who you are, why can't you accept me?"* it's the same thing as not being able to accept their nonacceptance. Wishing that our partners didn't need us to change is the same thing as wishing that they could change to be more like what we define as "better" or "good."

Sometimes, when Yuri gets upset about something, I find myself wanting to tell him, "Don't take it so personally." However, if I'm bothered or upset about it, it means that *I* am taking it personally that he's taking it personally.

So why don't *I* work on not taking it personally, as opposed to telling him to work on it?

In order to communicate better, it's not about me telling him not to be upset, it's about *me* not being upset that he is upset, because otherwise it's just the pot calling the kettle black and a never-ending cycle of upset-ness.

When you think about it, between two people, someone has to practice patience and maturity—so why are we always thinking that *the other person* should be less upset and more calm, when in reality *we* can practice those same qualities? Someone has to change, so why do we always want the other person to change?

No matter how tempting it is to want to push the work onto someone else, the truth is that it always comes back to us. It's *our* work, work that we cannot escape if we want to be happy.

If you don't think you hold onto the concept of fairness in your relationship but you are bothered and upset that your partner does, then it is an indication that you are actually also seeking fairness. Wanting someone to drop their ideals for yours is also a desire for fairness. It works both ways.

This goes for any negative charge we feel toward people. If someone is upset with us, it's not about telling them *not* to be upset, it's about us not being upset that they are upset.

In any communication between two people, it's never about who is more right, or who has more cause to be angry, or what is more fair. It's always about the difference in opinions, beliefs, and worldview, so it's about practicing the skills of being able to convey what is important to us while seeking to understand what the other person tell us is important to them. If we are busy being upset that they're wrong or that it's unfair, then we won't be able to listen well enough to understand.

And to think, "But I am doing all that! It's my partner who isn't listening or seeking to understand!" indicates that we *aren't* actually seeking to understand, because we can see that our frustration stems from our desire to be understood.

If we truly see the error of someone's behavior, and we truly believe that our own perspective is healthier, then it means that we are more capable in terms of maturity and wisdom, which means it is *all the more* imperative for us to practice understanding and patience.

We cannot dictate other people's actions, thoughts, and behavior, we can only decide on *our* own train of thought and response. If we hold onto being upset because we think we're right, it indicates that we are actually insisting that our partner change to adjust to us. Since the truth is that we have no power over our partner's actions, we are just going to get more and more frustrated.

Why waste all that effort into trying to change someone and end up being even more unhappy? Why don't we just turn all that effort to changing *ourselves*?

Again, when we put in the effort to be self-aware, understanding, and accepting, it's not for the other person, it's for *ourselves*. This is *our own practice*, and not something that we impose upon our partner as a thing they must also practice.

CREATING POSITIVE CHANGE REQUIRES US TO SEE THE BEST AND NOT THE WORST IN SOMEONE

<Acceptance>

A monk called Ajahn Brahm used to visit prisons where he would give classes to prisoners. It was found that the prisoners who went to his classes never returned to jail after they were released. Even Ajahn Brahm himself was surprised when the warden of the prison told him this and requested that he continue giving classes at the prison.

Ajahn Brahm pondered long and hard about why his classes produced such results. What did he do that genuinely reformed people—people who had committed serious crimes?

This was what he realized.

"I have seen a person who has murdered, but I have not seen a murderer."

"I have seen people who have stolen, but I've not seen a thief."

"I have seen people who committed terrible sex offenses, but I've not met a sex offender."

"I saw that the person was *more* than the crime."

This was a story I heard Ajahn Brahm tell in one of his talks. It really shows how the subtlest shift of our perspective can change the direction and result of an interaction.

When we label someone, then in our reality, that is the story of who they are—we are allowing no chance for the person to be anyone else but the role in the story into which we've painted them.

If you truly believe that your partner is a forgetful person, then you'll always feel upset whenever he or she forgets something; but being upset doesn't actually help them with their memory. It doesn't assist you in being loving, nor does it help the situation be a happy one. If anything, the story you have in your head about your partner is then cemented as a fact.

If it's already a fact to you, how can the person be anything else?

When we label someone—"My partner is a forgetful person"—two things happen.

The first is that we start to pay more attention to our partner's faults. We will absolutely notice *every time* they forget something, and we will be less likely to notice the times when they *do* remember. This will serve to make us more and more upset. The more upset we are, the more defensive or afraid the other person will be, resulting in less willingness or ability to change on their part.

The second is that our partners will tend to exhibit the undesirable characteristic more and more—people have a tendency to be *more* like who we *think* they are. If we see the best version of them, their best version will strive to emerge. If we see the worst version of someone, their worst self will strive to emerge.

We just have to look at students in schools to see evidence of this. Students put in "good" classes tend to flourish, and students put in "bad" classes tend to get worse. We are subtly yet strongly influenced by people's judgement of us. It is really hard to believe that you are worthy if you have had a teacher who has already labeled you as worthless.

And if kids can see through our judgements of them so easily, then what about everyone else on whom we have pronounced a judgement?

This is why it's so important for us to understand our own thoughts, and to discern the fine line between an opinion and a judgement. A child who is disrupting the class (opinion) isn't a "disruptive child" (judgement). A colleague who doesn't do their work well (opinion) isn't an "incompetent person" (judgement).

A partner who isn't able to give love the way we want (opinion) isn't an "selfish person" (judgement).

Most human beings can improve in one or more areas of their lives. The thing is, whether or not we change for the better depends a lot on who is teaching us. Similarly, if we want to exert positive influence on our partners, if we hope to help them or teach them better behaviors and ways of thinking and doing things, we have to decide on what approach to use in order to get the best results.

As in Ajahn Brahm's classes with the prisoners, it's not about how nice a person he was or how fierce a person he was. He didn't need to please the prisoners to get them to listen to him. He didn't have to threaten them and get them to fear him. He didn't need to use either the carrot or the stick—he used logic, understanding, and acceptance to lead them down the path of acknowledging for themselves the positive changes they needed to make in their lives.

TO HELP SOMEONE CHANGE, WE MUST GENUINELY ACCEPT THEM

<Acceptance>

One of the frequently asked questions I get is, "My partner is narcissistic, what do I do?"

To know the answer to this, we have to understand how we perceive our partner, and not labeling the person as a narcissist is a great place to start. Someone can certainly be self-absorbed or exhibit selfish behaviors. However, the challenge isn't how to "fix a narcissist," the challenge is in understanding *why* they are the way they are, so that we can help them be more aware and considerate.

A good question to ask is: If you have already labeled your partner as narcissistic and you believe that is the truth of who they are, then why are you with such a person?

Love is not a good reason, because to love someone is to accept a person without a strong judgement of who they are and who they should be.

Sometimes, we truly believe that our partner can benefit from positive change—that their potential for happiness and greatness would be so much better if they would do a little bit of this and a little bit of that. However, even if we can see that change is good for someone, the honest truth is that we cannot *make* someone change, we can only *inspire* them to want to change and then *support* them through their process of acting on their own desire to change.

If we choose to believe that a partner is a narcissist, it means that either subconsciously or consciously, we think that there is "something wrong" with them. So what happens is that even when we try to be patient, kind, and loving, our frustrations will come across and nothing gets better. This is because labeling someone doesn't encourage us to help the person change, it just propels us to try to "fix" the person. This is where we are unintentionally judging someone, because people only want to fix something when there's a problem, which indicates that *we think our partner is a problem*; and that's a judgement they can *feel*.

The only way to positively influence someone is to completely accept them for who they are. Again, accepting someone does not mean we are automatically applauding or approving of their actions, it means we are able to talk and communicate with the person without judging or labeling them.

Not judging or labeling someone is the first step to helping that person, because then our efforts are geared toward helping them improve their own lives instead of imposing on them what we think they should improve or change—it serves the person instead of serving our own needs. The mindset that works isn't to "fix" the person because something is wrong with them, it's to help the person enhance their quality of life.

Earlier in the book, I shared with you how my friend Mikayla believed in recycling while her boyfriend did not. She didn't want to impose her belief on him and therefore chose not to be upset or argue with him about the benefits of recycling.

Fast-forward a few years; Mikayla and I had another conversation about this incident. Something had happened—her boyfriend had gone over to his parent's house of his own accord to set up recycling bins for them!

When he was attempting to teach his parents how to recycle, he had to deal with the same protests that he himself had previously made a while before—*"But why is this necessary? How do you know the garbage collectors will recycle them accordingly?"*—and he patiently explained it all to his parents.

When Mikayla was telling me this story, we were both laughing. It is ironic how life gives us exactly what we want when we have no expectations!

Recycling had been important to Mikayla all along, so she most definitely preferred for her boyfriend to also believe in recycling.

However, she also did not judge him for *not* subscribing to what she thought was a good thing to do. Because there was no judgement, he wasn't defensive—and he also had very little resistance to exploring the idea of recycling on his own. What happened was that as he watched her recycle, he felt *inspired* to adopt the same habits. In the end, he recycled because he *wanted* to do so, and that resulted in true change.

For someone to change their belief or alter their worldview, they *themselves* have to see why it benefits them.

Often, we want people to change or to tweak aspects of themselves to improve. However, it is impossible to force change on someone. If Mikayla had gotten upset at her boyfriend and they had argued over it, he might have resisted the idea as a matter of pride and principle or because he felt upset that she couldn't understand his point of view. Or, he might have agreed to recycle because he wanted to make her happy or because he feared making her angry. But would he have *changed*? No. He would have just put in the effort without believing in it, or might even have felt frustrated or resentful that he was expected to do it.

Most of us do what our partner think we should do without really believing in it, but we do it to avoid an argument or problems in the relationship. This is why we can love someone yet slowly come to resent them, because there is a lot of fear that is mixed in with that love.

For people to even consider our ideas, we have to first drop our own ideas of how they should be.

Mikayla was able to do that because she didn't *need* for him to agree with her or share the same beliefs just because they are in a relationship. She was recycling happily before he came along, and she happily continued doing it regardless of whether he did it too. By doing so, she embodies someone who is truly confident from the inside—she doesn't need people to validate her beliefs in order to feel loved or recognized. She could disagree with her partner, yet not judge him.

This is the kind of acceptance where people who love us inspire us to be better versions of ourselves, because in their complete lack of expectations of who they need us to be, they help us to clearly see what we want to change about ourselves. When we feel like we need to measure up or to be better at something because we want to avoid disappointing the person we love, it is much harder to change for the better, because it's hard to change when it's not a change for ourselves, but for other people.

It feels paradoxical, yet it makes so much sense—to help someone change, we must first genuinely accept them. When there are no labels and no judgement, there is only logic, sense, compassion, kindness, and patience—all of which are tools to helping someone change positively, rather than merely wanting them to change so that *we* will feel better.

The reason why this is so important is because defensiveness and an unwillingness to listen are often barriers to positive change. So the objective isn't for us to impose our opinions upon our partner—no matter how right we think we are—the objective is for him or her to be open enough to think about what we say.

It's illogical to try incite positive change with negative methods. *"Girl, it's better to catch flies with honey,"* my mom used to tell me. If we want to positively influence someone, it is far more effective to draw them into it with positive motivation as opposed to giving them something unpleasant to dread. We want our partners to trust and respect us, because then they'll *want* to listen to us.

In order for us to incite any kind of change in others, we must first work on being able to let go of our own expectations, judgements, and resentment toward them. When we practice this in our personal relationships or apply this in our leadership roles, it transforms the way we interact with the people we love and with our colleagues at work.

TO CREATE POSITIVE
CHANGE, CHANGE YOURSELF

<Awareness>

When we are working on ourselves, there's often a strong desire to want the other person in our life to also work on themself. We might think that it's only fair to expect that, or maybe we feel that our unhappiness is not because we're not working on ourselves but because the other person is making it so hard for us.

However, no matter how justified or right we are, we cannot deny that wanting someone to be different from who they are always leads back to us wanting to *change someone else*.

When we read or listen to something inspiring, it is normal to wish that our partner, or our colleague, or our sister, or our mother-in-law can *also* read or listen to the same thing. We wish for them to have the same insights and realizations that we have so that they, too, can work on their own expectations and judgements. Because if they don't, it's hard for us, and it's incredibly frustrating to communicate with someone who is negative, critical, arrogant, narcissistic, or easily upset.

This is why relationships with people can be so difficult, because even if we try very hard each time to be patient and calm, it can easily go sideways when the *other person* is not practicing the same thing—and we feel like we really are trying or that we have genuinely tried, so it's easy to conclude that it is the other person not responding in kind that is the source of the problem.

The thing is, everyone has different levels of self-awareness and emotional maturity. Even members of the same family don't all share the same mindset nor the same strengths or skills. We might find talking to certain family members really difficult because of their narrow worldview, while we may find it refreshing to talk

to some other family members because they are open-minded
and introspective.

It can be frustrating when you notice that the person you're
talking to is lacking in self-awareness or the capacity to reflect and
grow; and it is at this point that it helps to remind yourself what
your objective is—to work on *yourself*, not for you to work on the
other person.

When we really look at what bothers us, we will often realize that
we have to implement in our own lives what we wish someone else
would practice in theirs. When we wish that a person were less
egotistical, all we have to do is look inwards to realize that our
dissatisfaction with the person is also coming from *our own* ego.

We'll only tell someone not to be so angry when we ourselves
are angry that they're angry. It doesn't matter who is right or
who is wrong, what matters more is *our own* reaction to what
is happening. No matter how we want to push the work onto
someone else, it always comes back to our own inner selves.

If we love someone yet we need them to change, it is time to
examine if we do indeed love the person or if it's actually that we
want or need them to fill the gaps in our lives.

If we keep being negatively affected by a family member or friend
and we need them to change, it is time to work on our own
triggers and take responsibility for our own happiness.

The truth is, we only have power over our own lives. We cannot
wait for other people to change. We cannot change only if *they*
change, because then our growth and progress as human beings
will be forever at the mercy of another person. We change because
we want to change, for ourselves.

Even when we focus all our energy into changing someone, it still
won't work out the way we wish it would. It is only when we
focus all our energy into being more self-aware and emotionally
mature ourselves that things start to change. The best way to bring
about positive change in a relationship isn't about fairness or
equality—it's about changing ourselves.

When you change—for yourself, and not with expectations of how the other person should also change—*everything* will start to change. Either the people around you will be *inspired* to change, or you'll find yourself growing as a person. Often, it is *because* you are growing in positivity and wisdom that the people around you are inspired to follow suit. This is because when we change ourselves and grow as human beings, our circle of positive influence grows wider and people start responding to us differently.

When we focus on changing others, we don't have enough energy to work on ourselves and we regress as a person—our circle of negative influence spreads, and that's why our relationships get worse instead of better.

In life, we try to be nice and we put a lot of effort into being smart, but creating positive change isn't about whether we are a nice or smart person—how we influence others is a result of how we view the world, how aware we are of ourselves, and how maturely or immaturely we communicate when problems arise.

We don't need to try to positively influence people, because when we are growing, it is something that naturally happens. The reward, however, doesn't come from having successfully changed people, it's from looking back and seeing how much we ourselves have grown.

One day, we might even wake up and be pleasantly surprised at how we don't need people to change anymore, and we'll realized that it's because *we* have changed—we may have learned how to be happy in our relationships, imperfect as they are.

Or we might find the courage to exit a relationship that isn't healthy for us, because we no longer need someone else to fill the gaps in our lives.

Or we might find ourselves being more compassionate and less affected by negative people because we don't depend on people to make us feel good about ourselves anymore.

Either way, we win.

CHAPTER THREE

Communicating Positively with Difficult People

IT'S NOT ABOUT NEGATIVE
PEOPLE, IT'S ABOUT NOT
BEING NEGATIVELY AFFECTED

<Understanding>

In life, it is a certainty that we will meet people whom we find difficult or challenging to handle. Sometimes, it's people at work or strangers we meet who upset us. Other times, it is our own family and friends who challenge us—they can push our buttons and test us with the things they say and do.

This is why it's so important for us to know what our buttons are so that we don't constantly allow people to trigger us so easily. Our real challenge isn't "difficult people," it is our own reactions and responses, which can keep us from communicating in a way that creates more happiness and less suffering for ourselves.

When people challenge our self-worth and treat us with less respect than we think we deserve, do we have strong enough self-esteem to understand that it has nothing to do with us, or do we take it personally and allow them to push our buttons?

It's very hard to remain calm and not be upset when people push our buttons, but no matter how we blame people for being difficult—even when it's absolutely their fault—we still cannot deny the fact that if we don't have buttons for people to push, they won't have the power to "make" us so upset.

This is why it's important to remember that whose fault it is isn't as important as how we move forward, because who is to blame depends on whose perspective we are seeing the situation from— nobody is a villain in their own story, so it's futile to let ourselves become too focused on blaming someone for being at fault.

People can definitely create difficult problems for us, but they cannot push our buttons if we work on not being sensitive and reactive. And this is something that only we can do for ourselves—nobody else can help us remove the barriers to our own happiness.

It has never been about how we can change or control someone who is being difficult, it is about how we can *respond* in a way that doesn't create more suffering for us. This is why, when we have to interact with someone who bothers us, it's less about asking the person, *"Why are you so negative?"* and more about noticing what's going on and asking ourselves, *"Why am I so negatively affected by you?"*

When we are facing a difficult situation with someone, it may already be painful, and being upset and resentful only serves to *add another layer* of suffering to our pain. If we constantly allow people to get to us so easily, we will constantly and easily suffer.

When things happen, the goal is always to focus on *what action to take*, and we will always have a better chance of figuring out a way to do that without the added layer of emotional suffering that plagues us if we don't understand ourselves and what our triggers are. It's not about controlling our emotions, but learning to acknowledge how we feel so that we can better understand ourselves.

This is why in this chapter, we will focus on how to *respond* positively instead of reacting negatively, even when it's challenging.

First, we will be examining if our thoughts and beliefs are creating more suffering for us—whether how we think is helping us or sabotaging us. As the chapter progresses, we will look at understanding our self-esteem and ego better so that we can better identify our triggers and sensitivities.

All of this leads to a better understanding of ourselves, so that even if people hurt us or take advantage of us, we can stand up for ourselves in a way that is gracious, strong, and emotionally mature. When we encounter a difficult interpersonal situation, we want to first understand our own reaction so that we can approach the situation with self-awareness and respond with emotional resilience.

Our happiness isn't dependent on who or what happens, but rather on how we respond that can bring about a positive outcome.

WHEN THE GOING GETS TOUGH, HOW DO YOU RESPOND?

<Awareness>

There are very few things in life that are guaranteed outside of life and death, but there's one thing that we can definitely depend on in our lifetime on earth, and that is *problems*.

No matter how we try to escape from hurt, difficulties, and challenges, we are bound to experience them. As long as we cross paths with other human beings, we will experience discomfort or difficulty, mild to extreme, because no other human being is exactly the same as we are.

This is why when it comes to being happy, taking responsibility for our own requires us to have a level of emotional maturity and resilience. This is because when times are good and we have no challenges with other people, it's really easy to be happy, just like it's easy to be strong enough when all we're carrying is a very light weight. It's when times aren't good and people are challenging us when we get to see how emotionally mature and resilient we are.

For example, when we start dating someone and get along really well with them, it's wonderful. At this stage, we are seeing the person's humor, manners, social skills, and everything that makes up their personality. This is when we usually determine if this is a person with whom we are compatible. Maybe we're even falling in love. And it is at this point that we want to better understand the *character* of this person. How do they react when things go wrong? How do they respond when people don't agree with them? How do they communicate when it's not easy?

In other words, at what level is this person's emotional maturity and resilience? And as we examine this, we turn the question inward—at what level is *my* emotional maturity and resilience? When the going gets tough, how do *I* respond? What is my level of awareness in terms of my triggers, sensitivities, and ego? Do I know what holds me back from being happy? Am I able to communicate and solve problems with patience and kindness, or do I often get carried away by my righteous anger? Do I know how to not outsource my happiness to other people even when they have hurt or wronged me?

Growing up, our schooling and our conditioning teach us how to be confident, mature, and intelligent people so we can carry on a conversation, make important decisions, and build ourselves a good career and a loving family.

Technically, because we put in so much effort toward living well, one would think we should be living our best life. However, being emotionally mature in responding to problems isn't something that is usually taught to us, and being emotionally resilient when navigating challenges isn't a skill that we automatically develop just because we get older.

We may have a great life, but to be able to *live* a great life requires a different set of skills.

We can be smart, but it is necessary to know the difference between intelligence and wisdom.

We can be confident, but it is even more important to have healthy self-esteem.

We may be physically capable, but our happiness depends on our emotional resilience.

When people are difficult and negative, do we have the wisdom to take responsibility for our happiness, or do we push that responsibility onto someone else by blaming them for our unhappiness?

Like our skills in music or sports, emotional maturity and resilience are something we have to consciously practice, and each time we encounter someone we find difficult, it is the perfect *opportunity* for us to practice.

DO PEOPLE MAKE YOU UNHAPPY? OR IS YOUR BELIEF MAKING YOU UNHAPPY?

<Awareness>

Some time ago, I watched a video of a woman sitting in her car, filming herself relating what had just happened at her local grocery store. She said that the checkout counter lines were longer than usual because the checkout boy was incredibly slow. He was fumbling and making mistakes and, as you can imagine, people started to get impatient. Impatience turned into tension, and someone lost their temper and started yelling at him in front of everyone for being so slow.

In her video, the woman narrated that the teenage boy tried to pull it together but instead broke down in tears. He was still trying to get people's groceries packed while he apologized, saying, "I'm so sorry, my mom committed suicide last night and I had to come to work because we need the money."

The woman went on to describe the reaction of the people in line. Immediately, there was a change in the air. She could feel that instead of being impatient, people suddenly didn't mind the wait.

Why would their behavior suddenly change? They were in the exact same situation that they had been in just a minute ago. They were still stuck in the line—needing to get out of the grocery store as soon as possible, some even late for work because of the unexpected delay—and the situation had not changed one bit, but their *attitude* toward the boy had changed.

Earlier, their underlying beliefs were likely to have been, *"What an idiot"* or *"He's so incompetent."* But once people heard what the teenager had to say, their beliefs likely changed to *"What a poor boy,"* or *"He's so strong."*

For the shoppers at that grocery store, nothing had changed, yet everything had changed.

This is the power of our thoughts—specifically, what we *believe* to be true.

When we get upset and agitated with someone, it is because we have a certain belief about who the person is. When we feel negatively affected, we have to ask ourselves, "Hang on...is this person making me unhappy, or is my *belief* about this person making me unhappy?"

When someone shoves you out of the way as you're walking on the street, you might believe that he's an uncouth, awful person. But if you were to find out that he shoved you out of the way to save someone from getting run over by a car, you'd believe that he's a brave and kind person. One belief makes you feel terribly angry, and the other belief makes you feel incredibly inspired. Our beliefs about someone can change so rapidly; this demonstrates to us how there is never one absolute truth.

The teenage boy at the supermarket happened to tell his story, thereby giving us a little insight into the reason behind his behavior. But how often do we get the chance to know the story behind someone's thoughts and actions? And if we don't know, why would we choose to believe the *worst* of someone, especially when that belief causes us so much unpleasantness and suffering?

WHEN WE UNINTENTIONALLY JUDGE PEOPLE, WE END UP UNINTENTIONALLY UNHAPPY

<Awareness>

One of the main reasons why it's so hard to let go of our negative feelings toward someone is because we have such a strong belief about who the person is.

When we notice someone's flaws, we instinctively judge the person by what we see. Yet most of us don't intentionally judge people. Ironically, our judgements of others often arise from our genuine intent to spread goodness. When we observe our thought patterns, we start to notice how our judgements of people stem from our own worldview of what is "good" and "right." These judgements then tend to harden into expectations of how we think people should be and lead to us labeling others or putting them into a box. If we're not aware of this, we will not be able to figure out that the reason why we are getting so upset at someone is because we are carrying a subconscious judgement of them.

One of the most important things to remember is that a human being is never one dimensional. We are made up of so many characteristics and emotions that to label ourselves as just *one* thing isn't accurate.

We have all been angry, rude, in a bad mood, or impatient at some points in our life—sometimes even several times in one day!—and we really don't want people to label us based only on *those* interactions. Because you're not an angry person, you were just angry over a particular situation. You're not a rude person, you were just in a bad mood that day. People may see you before you've had our morning coffee and categorize you as a "grumpy person," or they might see your impatience during work and categorize you as an "unhelpful person." They don't see and don't know that we are often also giving or kind or cheerful people.

When you look at it this way, it's not that it's *unfair* for people to judge us, it's that it *doesn't make sense* for people to judge us. When you turn the lens around, it is also equally impossible for us to judge other people. When we judge people based on *our own* reality and our limited information on them, it isn't an accurate representation of who they really are.

Sometimes, we think we know someone pretty well. We think that the information we have paints an accurate picture of who they are. These are the times when we feel even more adamant that the person is deserving of our anger and even hate. Still, is it really that easy to know the entirety of who a person is?

When you look at yourself and you try to unearth all the reasons why you would feel insecure, or identify your fears and needs, you might find it difficult to know and understand yourself. Often, we find that we don't actually know *why* we seem to behave and react the way we do—it's already so hard to know the absolute truth of who *we* are, much less know the absolute truth of who *someone else* is.

When we go about our daily lives, it is impossible to know the story of every single person we come across. Often, we don't even know what has happened in the lives of our family members, best friends, lovers, and partners—what were the experiences that shaped them when they were growing up?

All of us are shaped by our conditioning and experiences, all of which explain why people react the way they do when faced with challenges. Some people react negatively and some people respond positively. People are who they are because of what they've experienced since the day they were born.

Likewise, we are who we are because of what we've experienced in childhood. If someone judged us based on one part of our story, we might find it unfair. So why would we cement our belief of someone else when we don't know all the other aspects of their story?

When people do something we don't understand, it is our opinion about who they are that leads us to our suffering—indignation, anger, and hatred are all emotions that create more misery for us. In order to lift this layer of suffering, we have to be able to *change our beliefs* about the person or the situaion.

When we are interacting with another human being, we don't actually have any idea of the reasoning behind their reactions and responses—when someone is being mean, we usually don't know why. When someone is being rude, the rudeness is all we can see—we can't see the *source* of the rudeness in that person's life experiences, and because we cannot see it, we cannot understand it.

This is why changing our beliefs about people requires us to cultivate the practice of *understanding* people, because where there is understanding, judgement and resentment automatically fall away.

THE PERSON IS NOT DIFFICULT; THE PERSON IS JUST VERY DIFFERENT FROM YOU

<Understanding>

To help us understand people better, we have to first examine if our own perceptions and mindset are holding us back.

When we have to interact with someone difficult, these are two of the most important questions to ask ourselves: is *the person* difficult? Or do *I find* the person difficult?

Which is more true?

When you think about it, this "difficult person" has family and friends who don't find them difficult at all—in fact, they like and enjoy the company of this person. This is why when we find it incredibly difficult to talk to someone, deal with them at work, or be nice to that person, it's very important for us to understand *why* we think they're difficult.

In order to address a difficult situation with people, we have to first understand our own beliefs and perceptions about them—do we keep thinking that someone is difficult because we don't realize that we are projecting our own expectations on that person?

Before we proceed, it may help to refer back to the topic *"Your Normal Is Not the Universal Normal"* from chapter two. If you have not yet read chapter two, it'd be helpful to first do that before you continue with this, as the next chapter examines the concepts and practices that we discussed in that chapter more deeply.

You and I; we each have our own standards in life. These standards are made up of our ideals, values, and beliefs—they are the guiding principles for how we want to live our lives. Naturally, we all *believe* that our own standards are good, otherwise we wouldn't subscribe to them. This is why it's instinctive for us to assume that our standards are also *universal* standards and that our definitions of what is "right" and "good" are definitions that are universally embraced.

However, every single person who lives in this world has their *own reality* with their *own* standards and guiding principles, some of which may overlap with ours (by which I mean that they have similar standards and principles) and some of which may have absolute *no* overlap with our reality (meaning that they have very different standards and principles).

This why when we happen to meet people whose guiding principles don't overlap with our own, we may be shocked, offended, insulted, and upset over their behavior.

Referring back to the Expectation Circle 1.3 graphic from chapter two (shown below), we can see that some people's realities lie so far away from our own reality that talking to them is like talking to someone from another planet—they are like aliens to us!

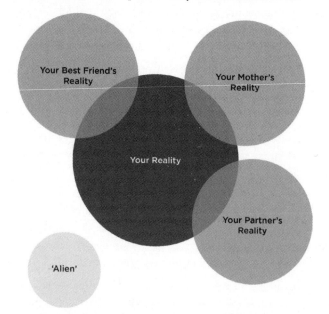

The Expectation Circle 1.3: Your relationship with people

Most of the people we like and love—our good friends and family—also subscribe to similar standards and guiding principles. Their realities are so close together that they overlap with ours, which further strengthens how we experience our ideals, beliefs, and values as "correct" and "normal."

For example, if everyone in your family defines "respect" as "never arguing with your elders," it's only natural that if your subordinates or interns at work question your decision-making, you'll find them incredibly disrespectful and rude and the entire situation unacceptable.

However, taking another look at Expectation Circle 1.4, we can see that working from the reality of the "alien"—from the other person's point of view—*you* are the alien. You are so far apart from their reality that *they* might think *you* are difficult, impossible, crazy, unfair, and/or incompetent.

That person, too, has family and friends who share a similar worldview, set of beliefs, ideals, and principles, so they also feel validated and justified in their own behavior, just as you do. So in their reality, *you* are foreign and difficult to understand.

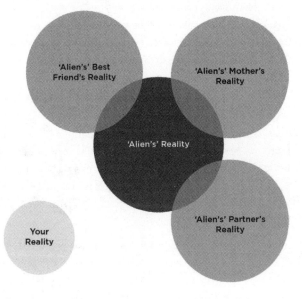

The Expectation Circle 1.4: The alien's point of view

The reason I call it "Reality" in the Expectations Circle and not simply "Perspective" is because it's important for us to understand that what people believe in is *real* to them. Similarly, what we believe in is very real to us—we object to anyone who challenges the validity of our reality, which is precisely why we would categorize some people as "difficult."

This is why it's really hard for human beings to understand other human beings who are very different, because it's extremely difficult for us to change what we believe is *real*. It's not just changing our minds—it's changing what we consider to be real. Similarly, we can have a difficult time with other people's perspective and behavior because it's hard for them to change what they consider real.

Understanding this is already a form of acceptance, because when people rub us the wrong way, we can see that it is our *differing standards and beliefs* that are creating the friction, not *the person*.

People are difficult to deal with because they are *different* from us. The form of acceptance described here does not mean that we have to agree with them. Accepting someone for who they are doesn't mean we approve of their actions or respect their decisions. What it does mean is that we stop blaming people and defining them as the source of our problems. When we have a difficult time communicating or interacting with someone, our problem isn't actually *the person,* our problem is the anger or resentment we feel toward that individual, which stops us from being able to communicate effectively with them.

People can create a multitude of difficult situations for us, but they cannot *make us* feel upset or unhappy. Our happiness and our emotions have never belonged to other people, and when we *blame* someone just for being who they are, it means we are giving our power away to them by constantly *reacting* to what they have "done to us."

People are not usually trying to offend us or sabotage us. If they are offensive or unscrupulous, it definitely *feels* very personal. However, it really helps us to suffer less when we understand that it's *not* personal—people are just behaving in accordance with the norms in their own reality. There really is no point getting upset over thoughts like, *"But he or she should have known better,"* because *how* would they know better?

People only know what they know from their own reality, and they are not aware of what they don't know. Understanding this does not mean we excuse people's rude or bad behavior, but it does mean we can *approach the situation* without getting all upset over it. If we keep getting upset over "difficult people," it just feeds our ego by making us feel justified for reacting badly. However, if we can see the logic of how people are just very diverse with extremely different standards, beliefs, and ideals, we can *understand* that they are just behaving in accordance to what is "normal" in their own reality.

When we are able to let go of the concept of "should," we stop projecting the norms in our reality on other people. This way, we *see* people for who they are without being upset that they are not "more like us." Because the truth is that there are many people in this world who are not like us.

Some people are just in our lives—we can't choose our family members, much less our colleagues at work. If you *have* to see someone you don't like and you must interact with him or her, it becomes even more important to drop your expectations and then your judgements of this person.

If you don't, you will constantly benchmark what they say or do against what *you* would say or do—*"If I were her, I wouldn't say that!"*—and it will result in you constantly feeling hurt, miserable, or angry. This is self-imposed pain, because the truth is, you are *not* that person, so to keep comparing their actions to what you would or wouldn't do in their shoes doesn't make sense.

Putting ourselves into someone else's shoes is not thinking, "If I were you, I would have done things differently." Empathy is understanding that if we were in someone else's shoes, that means we would *also walk like them*—not just wear their shoes and still walk like ourselves.

If we had been born in that person's position, had experienced exactly what they experienced, and had the same needs and fears that they have, then we would behave *exactly* like that person—this is what it means to walk in someone else's shoes, and this is the understanding that empathy brings.

This understanding leads to being able to not be angry or resentful when we are interacting with someone who is very different, because we have accepted that people are who they are and we don't keep *expecting* the person to behave the same way *we* would behave.

When we stop seeing people as difficult, they cease to be difficult. It's not that they have changed—they are still the exact same people, with the exact same attitudes and character traits—but that *we* have changed. When our beliefs change, the way we respond also changes.

If our belief is that people are "difficult," then it's very hard for us to let go of our negative emotions toward them, because there is a lot of blame involved. If our belief is that people are "different," then it's easier for us to disagree with someone without suffering, because there is understanding involved.

This doesn't mean we allow people to walk all over us—because it's very important that we address the problem or the situation— but it does mean that we are able to be free of frustration and negativity when communicating with someone we find difficult. This is what it means to not be triggered by people.

We lift away this first layer of suffering so that we can better face the challenges before us.

When we don't blame people for how we feel, we stop outsourcing our happiness to them so easily. This is true freedom, and it allows us to move forward and take action without people holding our happiness hostage.

IF YOU EXPECT A DOG TO MEOW, YOU'RE DEFINITELY GOING TO BE DISAPPOINTED!

<Acceptance>

When I was working at a radio station, there were times when I would come home incredibly upset at the way certain people worked. And there was one guy in particular who would say and do things that just did not make sense to me, and I would come home and unleash all my pent-up frustration by venting about him to my mom and Yuri.

During one of my venting sessions, Yuri could see how affected I was, and he said, "A dog will bark and a cat will meow. If you expect a dog to meow, then you're always going to be let down."

I burst out laughing mid-vent when I heard that. It sounded funny, the animal comparison, but it did hold incredible wisdom. What he said was *true*. As human beings, we are all always going to behave in accord with how we usually behave—people are merely who they are, so if we keep getting frustrated at how they behave, it's not even close to logical.

If we keep expecting the dog to meow...then we're not being logical.

I realized how silly it was that I would get frustrated *every time* this guy did something I didn't think was right—why I was *allowing* this one person to affect me so much? I had to stop complaining and really examine the possibility that perhaps *he* wasn't the problem. Maybe it was the way I was approaching the whole situation that was making it a problem for me.

Looking inward is always less fun than looking at other people. And even when we examine our inner selves, we may not be entirely honest about why we feel the negative feelings that we do.

This is why I've developed a way of questioning myself that helps lead me to answers that allow me to be as honest with myself as possible, thereby allowing me to be as *happy* as possible. I call it "Two-Layer Reasoning."

The first layer of reasoning is the *surface* reason why we're upset—this is the most immediate answer that comes to us when someone affects us negatively. In my case, my Surface-Layer Reasoning answer was, "I'm upset because this person isn't good at his job and it reflects negatively on the whole team!"

The second layer is the *deeper* reason why we're upset—it is the answer that relates more to *us* than to the *other person* when someone affects us negatively. My Deeper-Layer Reasoning led me down a different path.

People only upset us when they behave in a way that is *unexpected* to us. This person was in a leadership position, and I had expectations of how he *should* behave as a leader. Instead of accepting him for who he was, I was fighting the reality of his actual self.

We often think that accepting people for who they are means we are subscribing to what is against our own beliefs, but acceptance of who people are doesn't mean we're automatically condoning their actions—it's just us releasing ourselves from wanting or needing a person to be someone they're not. This was so crucial for me to understand, because I hadn't realized that I was continually frustrated because I kept thinking he *should* be different, but the *reality* is that he is who he is. No matter how unaccepting I was or how upset I got, he was *still* going to be the exact same person. So if I refused to accept him and kept insisting on measuring him against my own standards of what good leadership ought to be, I would continue to create my own suffering.

The other thing I realized was that we can have a *strong opinion* about someone without it being a judgement—I had the opinion that he wasn't good at his job and that it was affecting the team, but I realized that I could still strategize on working around his ineffectiveness *without* all the angst and anger that came from judging him. The moment I let go of my judgement of him and who he "should be," it became so much easier to not continually be upset over everything he said or did.

When I went deeper into my second-layer reasoning of why I was being so negatively affected, I also realized that it was a matter of pride. When I kept highlighting his inadequacy, it was inadvertently highlighting my own competency, and I think doing that gave me a sense of validation and pride.

When you think about it, this is why complaining and venting about people feels so rewarding. If you notice, every time we talk about how people are incompetent or stupid, it is like waving a flag to highlight how *we are so much better*. It gives us a sense of validation to complain about people, because in a way, it showcases our own goodness and superiority. If we have something to say about someone, it means that we think we are better at that particular thing. When we say, *"She's so unprofessional!"* we are also indicating, *"I am professional."*

This awareness was harder to come by. I only noticed this when I asked myself *why* complaining and venting made me feel better. When I became aware that it was my pride—and that therefore, my ego was involved—I realized that I could still talk about my feelings about this person *without* the emotional charge that came with it. When I stopped letting my ego drive my actions, talking about this guy at work stopped being a venting or complaining session and became rather just a sharing of facts of what had happened at work.

Sometimes, it is the smallest changes in the way we perceive something that make the most difference to how much emotional suffering we experience.

WHEN TWO PEOPLE
DISAGREE, WHO IS RIGHT?

<Perspective>

We all understand that every single person is different, yet this understanding can quite easily vanish into thin air the moment we interact with someone who is *actually different* from us.

We don't think that we're always right, but we do believe in truths and realities, so we tend to believe that between two people, someone has to be right and someone has to be wrong. And when we believe vehemently that someone is wrong, it can be very difficult for us to let go of self-righteous anger, which is one layer of suffering that weighs us down.

If you see a tree in front of you and a blind man tells you it's not there, who is right and who is wrong? Which reality is the real reality?

For people who have vision, we assume that we all see the same thing. But although our eyes may capture the same image, the way we *interpret* those visual signals can be extremely different. It is like how two people can look at the same photograph yet describe it completely differently.

When it comes to seeing something with our eyes, we may both have vision, but *what* we see depends on a multitude of factors.

In 2015, there was a debate about distinguishing the color of a dress in a photo that went viral on the internet. Some people said the dress was black and blue, and other people saw it as gold and white, but it was the exact same dress and picture!

My husband and I looked at it—he saw black and blue, while I saw gold and white. I remember being absolutely amazed at the science of how we could look at the *same thing* at the *same time* and yet see something completely *different*.

Then in 2018, an audio clip surfaced on the internet that caused an uproar worldwide. It was a computer-generated voice saying one word repeatedly—some people heard "Laurel," whereas others insisted that they heard "Yanny." Again, there was a huge and (and even heated) debate over it. My husband and I listened to the same recording, yet we heard something completely different! He heard "Laurel," while I clearly heard "Yanny." Later, he could hear both names, but I could still only hear "Yanny."

We had a great laugh—but if we were to base our relationship on the results of these two experiments, our marriage would be doomed to fail, because we literally could not see or hear something *so obvious* to the other!

This shines a light on how we as human beings perceive the world through our own individual lenses; but on the surface, we're not usually conscious of the different lenses through which people see the world—when something is obvious to us, we automatically assume that it should be obvious to the other person as well. Like, "Hey, it's obvious that the sky is blue." And if someone were to *argue* with you about the color of the sky, you'd be upset and filled with indignation, and you'd want to ask them, *"But how can you argue against reality?!"*

This is the main reason why we get increasingly frustrated when we try to explain our own concepts to people—we don't understand how they can keep denying something that is so obviously true!

This is fueled further by the fact that our family and friends share our point of view; we know people who agree with our perspective, our work ethic, and our principles, so in a way, we have proof and validation that our way of thinking and doing things is *right*.

However, we know that truths and realities often look different depending on the color of the lenses we wear. Both the visual and audio internet phenomena shine a light on the fact that how our brains see something is just the way our senses process it, it is *not the reality of the world*. Just because *more people* agree with us and our reality, it doesn't mean that we are "more right," just as if more people hear "Laurel" in an audio clip, it doesn't make it a more legitimate interpretation than "Yanny."

This is why the concepts of "right" and "wrong" are so futile in a difficult discussion. What seems normal to me may not be normal to you. We can argue until the end of our days, and all we'll achieve is a whole lot of frustration and resentment.

If the belief is "you are wrong," then it's very hard to communicate with the other person without getting emotionally riled up and triggered.

Right or wrong doesn't matter as much as what *action* we are going to take next to address the situation in a way that meets our own objectives. We don't want to be so caught up in feeling righteous that we serve the ego instead of serving our own objectives.

WHEN YOU CARE WHOSE FAULT IT IS, YOU CANNOT BE HAPPY

<Understanding>

When something goes wrong, as it inevitably will, who is at fault?

Are you at fault? Is the other person at fault? Or is circumstance at fault?

We usually think that we *must* know whose fault it is so that the person can take responsibility for fixing it, but the truth is, even when someone is *responsible* for causing a mess, for breaking our heart, for not doing their job well...blaming them doesn't mean they will take responsibility, and it certainly doesn't solve the problem.

There is a renowned designer in Malaysia, Bernard Chandran, who has five beautiful children with his wife Mary. They live in a magnificent home. Since Bernard works in fashion, he has impeccable taste in interior design and is a self-proclaimed neat freak. Whenever I visit their home at Christmas, I am blown away at how clean and sparkling every surface is. Their oldest son, Teri, went off to study in the United States, where he resided off campus with a few housemates.

"How is it, being away from home?" I asked him. "Must be exciting!"

"Yes, it's pretty great, but I don't like the living situation with my housemates. I can't stand being in the house! It's so dirty!" he shuddered.

His mom, who was sitting next to him, laughed.

"Don't you guys have a cleaning schedule?" I asked, not at all surprised by his distress at the lack of hygiene. It had to be hard to adjust to any place that was less than spic-and-span after being used to his parents' remarkably clean house.

"Yes, we do! But they don't clean when it's their turn! The toilet is absolutely disgusting!"

"Have you talked to your housemates about it? Maybe you can stress the whole hygiene thing?"

"I tried talking to them, but it doesn't work. They still don't clean because they don't see it as a problem at all."

"So what happens now?" I asked.

"So I have to clean the toilet all the time, because I can't even *look* at the toilet bowl in that state, much less use it." He said, looking terribly resigned, yet surprisingly accepting for someone who had to keep cleaning the toilet that *everyone* was using.

At this point, his mom quipped, "I told him that if he wants to use a clean toilet, then he should just clean it himself! It doesn't matter that it's a shared toilet. He'll feel more miserable always waiting for them to clean it than if he just cleaned it himself."

No one could argue with that logic! I loved how Mary wasn't jumping to defend her son on how unfair the whole situation was, but rather simply let him know that in life, you are responsible for your own happiness—and your own clean toilet.

So many of us have been in similar positions. Things are not fair, and we have to pick up the slack.

If you were in Teri's shoes, there would be a few options on what you could do. If you chose to continue living in the apartment— either because you didn't want to or couldn't move out—you would have these options:

    a.   Hold your breath every time you use the dirty toilet and be completely grossed out each time;

    b.   Drive to the nearest public toilet every time you need it;

    c. Clean the toilet angrily, and complain bitterly each time you do it; *or*

    d. Clean the toilet without thinking it's unfair because you understand that it is *your objective* to use a clean toilet.

Only one of the above actions is winning, because every other action would cause you more inconvenience or mental torture.

This understanding can help us in every aspect of life, especially at work or at home when we feel something is unfair. What may seem unfair on the surface—doing something even when it's not your job, or your turn, or your fault—is actually you meeting your own objective.

Sometimes we can completely lose sight of our main objective and sabotage ourselves just to prove a point, all while *mistakenly* thinking that blaming someone means we win (which is what the above options a, b, and care). There is a very big difference between satisfaction and happiness; we have to understand our ego enough to know the difference.

In life, sometimes it's really not your fault. In fact, sometimes, it is totally someone else's actions or behavior that have caused a negative situation or outcome. When this happens, don't ask yourself the question, *"Whose fault is it?"* but rather, *"What am I going to do that will create the most happiness for me?"*

It is always necessary to take *action*, it is never necessary to get hung up about whose fault it is.

DON'T LET THE CONCEPT OF FAIRNESS MAKE YOU LOSE SIGHT OF YOUR OBJECTIVES

<Understanding>

I receive many messages on my videos and live chats online, and a recurring problem faced by many is feeling that things are not fair.

There was a viewer who wrote in—let's call her Janice—to say that her boss had taken a liking to her new colleague because this colleague came across as very hardworking. Janice wasn't very happy about this because she felt that she had been contributing so much to the company over the years, yet her boss hadn't taken notice of her efforts as she had with this new co-worker.

One day, Janice decided to check the company's computer system to see what this co-worker had been so busy with at her desk, and lo and behold, she found that her co-worker was actually on Facebook when everyone else thought she was "busy working"!

This upset Janice even more, because now there was the added injustice of her boss mistakenly favoring this young woman who was probably less hardworking and lazier than Janice herself! This, she told me, was making her feel extremely demotivated, and she had no enthusiasm at work.

Janice had a choice of a few different actions that she could take, all of which depended on her *objective*.

If Janice's objective was to feel satisfied, and maybe to sabotage her coworker's career, she could choose to go to her boss and tell her boss about her coworker's Facebook activities.

If Janice's objective was to feel justified in hating her coworker and being angry at her boss, she could choose to continue going to work feeling demotivated and unenthusiastic.

If Janice's objective was to convey to her boss and everyone working at the company that she's hardworking and worthy of the next promotion, she could go to work with *more* enthusiasm and be *more* motivated to take the initiative to let her work and personality shine through.

Was Janice's colleague wrong to be on her Facebook at work? It is very likely that she was indeed breaking some rules at the company. However, was this *important* to Janice's objectives?

There are *many more* choices of action that Janice could have taken, but at no point did the concept of fairness enter the picture, because what mattered the most was, how was she going to get what she wanted? How could she meet her objectives?

If Janice's objective was to show that she was more hardworking and more deserving of recognition than her colleague, then going to work in a demotivated and unenthusiastic state would be self-sabotage. It's very rare indeed that a boss feels compelled to promote someone who comes to work grumpy and resentful.

When something happens, it's instinctive for us to immediately react. For Janice, feeling demotivated and going to work unenthusiastically wasn't something she planned to do—it was a reaction to what had happened.

This is why it's so important for us to first be really clear about what our objectives are, so that when things happen that upset us, we can act, not react.

If we're not clear about our objectives, what will often happen is that at every point of challenge and discomfort, we'll be reacting to the situation or the person instead of taking actions that can help bring us closer to the result we really want to achieve. It can be very easy for us to get caught up in the idea of what is "wrong" and react according to what we believe is "fair" without realizing that we're sabotaging our own goals.

Sometimes, we see our immediate need and think that it's our objective, but often, our real objective requires us to think a few steps further and consider the bigger picture. Needing someone to admit they're wrong or needing something to be fair may seem like a very important objective when we are angry with another person; but when we look further, we will often realize that our real objective in the big picture is to take action to address the situation or solve the problem in a way that causes the least suffering and brings about the most happiness.

In our careers, we have our career objectives.

In our relationships, we have our relationship objectives.

In our families, we have our family objectives.

In our lives, we have our life objectives.

Everyone's objectives differ, but there is an objective that most of us have in common, and that is to bring more happiness and less suffering into our lives. This is why when we allow people to make us miserable, we have to be mindful that we are taking ourselves further away from our own objective of being happy.

WHEN SOLVING PROBLEMS, ASK, "IS MY REACTION PART OF THE PROBLEM?"

<Awareness>

Sometimes, we think that if we don't react, people are going to take advantage of us!

This is why it's important to understand what a reaction is—a reaction is an immediate response to something based purely on instinct and emotional charge, usually with little or no thought given to the consequences or to our objectives. Simply put, we react when provoked.

Not reacting doesn't mean not taking action. It's important to act—and not react—when something is happening or has happened. A constructive action is a strategic and logical move that we execute based on what works best for our objectives in the situation, and most importantly, a move based on what brings the most happiness and the least suffering.

When we have difficulties with someone, we often attribute it to "miscommunication," but in truth, our difficult interactions with another person aren't so much about miscommunication as they are about the *emotions* that are at play. It is often the emotional charge that we bring into a discussion that creates a barrier to our good intentions and our positive actions.

Before we can communicate effectively, we have to first address our emotions and immediate reaction. We have to develop a clear focus on what objectives we're trying to achieve in any given communication.

For example, in customer service, there's a common saying, "The customer is always right." However, no one in this universe is always right—not our parents, not our teachers, not our partners, not us, nor all customers. If we work in customer service, the important thing to remember is that it's *not important* to spend our time trying to determine is the customer is right or wrong—what is more important is to understand that an undesirable situation has occurred and that our objective is to bring it to a better resolution.

Whether or not someone is being unreasonable, it is *up to us not to react*, but instead to take action to navigate the situation in a way likely to meet our objectives without our emotions clouding our judgement. If *we also* become unhappy in reaction to the other person's unhappiness, then there are *two* problems to be addressed—our own emotions as well as the situation at hand.

Often, when we are having trouble communicating with people, we get very caught up in who is right and who is wrong and who is to blame and who is at fault. We think that answering those questions (or getting the other party to admit they are wrong!) will help solve the problems we're facing with someone, but before we can even address a problem, we have to make sure our reaction does not *become part of the problem*.

The same thing applies to *any* difficult situation we face with people. In our relationships with our partners, family, friends, and colleagues, we can get so frustrated because we often get stuck at, "But *he (or she)'s the one* who has to be right all the time!"

Here's the funny thing—when we get upset at someone's need to be right, it is an indication that *we also* have a need to be right, because if we didn't have this need, we wouldn't be triggered by the person at all.

If we can see that a person's aggressiveness and unreasonableness comes from their ego, it doesn't make sense for us to get more angry at them, because the logical thing to do is to not bring *our own ego* into the situation.

When people react to what we say or do, it doesn't make sense for us to *react to their reaction*. No matter how other people behave, the way we respond to any challenging or difficult situation is always our choice.

This is essentially what is meant by self-awareness and emotional resilience. When it comes to communicating with someone we find difficult, it means that we are aware of how we feel and are able to listen to someone disagreeing with us without reacting badly. This is only possible when we understand ourselves enough—our ego and our objectives—that we can genuinely seek to understand someone even when they are behaving in a way we think is difficult or unreasonable.

It's important to take action when addressing a problem, and to do that we have to first not let our reaction become part of the problem.

TO BE UNDERSTOOD, WE HAVE TO FIRST UNDERSTAND

<Understanding>

When we are trying to communicate with someone, what is our objective?

Most of us would respond by saying, "I'm trying to address the issue and solve the problem." However, when we start to become emotionally charged, it's really easy to get derailed from talking about the issue at hand. How many times have we started a conversation with good intentions only to end up talking around in circles and losing sight of our objectives because we are too emotionally charged?

Often, we are not aware of the subconscious expectations that we carry into a conversation, and it is these expectations that make it so hard for us to communicate positively even when we are indeed making huge efforts to do so.

Very few people go into a conversation wanting to change someone, yet that is what most of us end up subconsciously trying to do. When we examine why we get emotionally charged and angry at the person with whom we're interacting, it's usually because we think that they *should not* be behaving the way they are behaving, that they *should not* be saying what they are saying, and that they *should not* be reacting the way they are reacting.

Without our even realizing it, the source of our negative reaction toward someone is that we keep projecting our expectations of how the person should be. This means that when we are upset, it is because we have a subconscious objective for the person to *change* from who they are into whom we would like them to be.

"You shouldn't say that!" means we want the person to change what they believe in.

"I wish you would understand!" means we want the person to change their mind.

Such an expectation in itself sabotages the way we communicate at the outset, because no matter how hard we try to be patient, calm, and kind, we are *already* carrying with us expectations and judgements of the person, which makes it really hard for us to not react negatively when the person doesn't give us the response we want.

If we truly understand that people are different, then we must be able to *allow* people to *be* different. If we truly believe that no one is perfect, then why do we get so upset when people show us their imperfections?

This is why accepting someone for who they are is so important and is key to communication, because then, we can talk to with someone who is difficult, negative, unreasonable, angry, and everything in between *without also* getting riled up. People are who they are. It helps to remember that if we keep expecting a dog to change its bark to a meow, then we are the ones being foolish.

Often, we go into a conversation with the objective that the other person must *understand us.* This is very much a subconscious intention, but when you examine why you would feel so upset when someone still doesn't understand despite you trying your best to present clear and logical points, you'll likely find that it's because you think the person *should* understand. This is why we often think, "But I already *told you!"* and then feel terribly frustrated when the other person still doesn't get it.

Our negative reactions often arise from the fact that we feel that we've already tried our best to explain, so it doesn't make sense that the other person isn't conceding or agreeing to what we're saying. This is why we get so upset when someone argues with us, because we have a belief that they shouldn't be this unreasonable!

It's not that we don't try our best at communication, but what often happens is that we end up just *telling* someone something. Communication is not about needing someone to understand us or needing them to agree with us, rather it is about being curious instead of getting upset when they don't understand or agree with us.

It sounds so simple, but it makes a world of difference when we're trying to communicate with someone we find difficult. Seeking to understand before needing to be understood means that we are simultaneously letting go of our expectations of how the other person should respond while being genuinely curious and interested in understanding the other person's reality, no matter how foreign it may seem to us.

Most of us try to prepare ourselves for a difficult conversation by focusing on patience and listening as our main objective, but it can be very hard to meet those objectives when we keep getting distracted by our own reactions.

Instead of just forcing ourselves to be patient and listen, we can *focus on the objective of seeking to understand* before needing to be understood, because then we will be less emotionally charged when people disagree with us or don't give us the response we want. It is like an emotional switch—we go from being upset to being genuinely curious about someone. This way, we are naturally more patient and able to listen better as a result.

It's important to note that seeking to understand is not about forcing ourselves to agree with opinions which we don't have common ground with—it's about being genuinely interested in understanding someone else's reality, however different it may be from our own.

When you find yourself feeling charged while interacting with someone you find difficult, whether it's your partner, mother in-law, colleague, friend, or even a stranger, remember that there is so much more to the person than you can see.

We don't know why people are the way they are, or why they think the thoughts they think, or why they treat people the way they do—we only know someone through the very narrow lens of what we understand of them, so it is wiser to choose a belief that causes us the *least* suffering.

We seek to understand someone not for the sake of that person but for ourselves, because only when our perspective and belief shifts can we let go of our negative emotions toward the person.

When people feel they are being listened to and sense that we are not passing judgement on them, they are naturally more receptive and open to listening when *we* speak. This is why we don't have to be afraid of "losing" when we listen to people, because seeking to first understand before needing to be understood helps lower people's barriers and defenses against us, which makes it easier for them to listen to us. At the same time, when we understand someone better, we can strategize to convey our messages in a way that we think *they can best accept*, instead of just telling the person the way *we want* to be understood. Conveying a message to someone in a way that they can accept and understand is a skill that can only be developed if we are willing to first seek to understand the person.

My mother is great at communicating with people others find difficult, because she has the patience to listen and approach the situation in a way that doesn't put people on the defensive. This is because when she talks to people, she naturally seeks to understand, and people can feel the lack of expectation and judgement. This is why one of the best pieces of advice my mom has given me when it comes to communication is to "not put someone on the defensive."

My mom has very little need to be understood, yet she *always* manages to convey her message, because she knows that when people are not on the defensive, they are already in a better frame of mind to better understand you.

The goal is never to merely please or placate someone, but to understand where they're coming from so we have enough insight and information on what steps to take next, and how to take those steps in a way that can help us meet our own objectives of resolving the problem or addressing the situation at hand.

WE DON'T NEED TO AGREE TO UNDERSTAND

<Understanding>

The thing is, understanding someone we don't agree with or that we don't even like or respect can be a very hard thing to do. This is why we have to first understand why we would even want to put in the effort to understand someone.

Since we cannot change someone we find difficult, we only have two options: to continue being negatively affected by them, or to change what we believe and feel toward the person so that we are not affected by them.

What usually happens, however, is that we choose a third option that lies somewhere in between, and that is to *try* not to be upset at the person and to *try* to be calm and patient; but despite our best efforts, we end up feeling more and more negatively affected.

This is why when we already feel frustrated at someone, we usually get *even more* frustrated, because we are putting in effort to change the way we feel, yet it doesn't yield the positive results we want.

At moments like these, it helps to examine if we are "trying our best" with judgement and resentment. If so, our unspoken frustration and silent anger will always come through as loud as any spoken language, which sabotages any efforts we're making.

I was once hosting an event with someone whose attitude and behavior I completely did not agree with. He was rude and egotistical, and I was trying very hard not to be affected because our dislike of each other might have come through onstage, which would not serve my objective of doing my best to serve the audience watching—it would be self-sabotage to let him affect me to the point of it affecting my job.

Even with this awareness, it was becoming increasingly difficult for me to be nice to him. It was then that I came to the realization that the work I had to put in shouldn't have been to be "nice," the work I had to put in was the practice of understanding.

When I started to seek to understand, I began to feel differently toward him—I still didn't agree with his behavior, but he stopped having so much power over my emotions. I genuinely wasn't upset with him because I had let go of any judgements and resentment toward him; and this was only possible because of my having made the choice to look at him from the perspective of understanding instead of frustration.

When we practice understanding someone we find difficult, we don't have to attempt to be patient, calm, or kind, because patience, calmness, and kindness will come as a *result*. It is natural that when we seek to understand someone, our minds will go down the path of curiosity instead of anger. We become *interested* instead of *angry* at why someone would behave the way they do.

When we try to understand someone, we catch glimpses of their needs and fears that come through, which tell us a lot about why they would be aggressive, rude, offensive, critical, or hateful.

It is the same practice as when we work to understand ourselves— when we are curious about our own actions and reactions, we will see that our defensiveness, indignation, irritation, frustration, anger, and hatred come from our own needs and fears.

This is why the practice of understanding people is one of the most amazing practices in life—because when we understand someone, our anger and hatred automatically drop away.

And here's the thing—when *we understand that we don't understand someone*, it also becomes impossible to hold on to anger or to hate the person, because how can we hate something or someone we don't understand?

When we understand that people are just different from us, we understand that their behavior toward us—any negativity, hostility, or aggression—stems from their own worldview, beliefs, and standards and has nothing to do *with us*.

In the case of my co-host, I was able to understand that although his attitude and behavior toward me felt very personal, it wasn't personal at all, so it was up to me to not take it personally and react to him. If I allowed myself to react to him, it would mean that I blamed him for my own suffering, and worse, that I would be allowing my reactions toward him to affect the quality of my job performance.

One of the main reasons we are so reluctant to understand others is because we feel we're allowing them to take advantage of us. However, understanding people isn't the same as giving them permission to walk all over us or treat us like a doormat—understanding means that we are not fighting against the reality of who they are.

Understanding that we *don't* understand someone brings a level of acceptance of the person—acceptance doesn't mean we approve, it just means we are not suffering by wishing things were different, because things are exactly as they are, and it is up to us to take action in a way that meets our own objectives.

People can indeed make things incredibly difficult for us, and moving forward, we need to address such situations *without* reacting negatively toward the person involved. Why would we want to allow people to cause us more suffering?

This sounds incredibly difficult—and it is, especially when the person has done something that has had a huge impact on our lives. However, no matter how difficult it may be, we still need to deal with each challenge in our lives. Whether or not we deal with it angrily or calmly, and whether or not we deal with it with stress or without stress, we *still* need to address such situations.

This is why the practice of seeking to understand someone doesn't mean that we are automatically agreeing with the person or condoning their actions. It just means that we can have a difficult interaction with someone without the concept of *should* making us so angry that we inevitably suffer.

DIFFICULT CONVERSATIONS NEED NOT BE A CONFRONTATION

<Understanding>

In life, there are many difficult and uncomfortable subjects we need to discuss with people. Even within families, there are difficult conversations that are part of the parent and child relationship. Most of us *avoid* difficult conversations because we see them as confrontational.

The very concept of confrontation is already scary—the word *confront* already implies a hostile or argumentative intent. One of the main reasons we may be so afraid or wary of a difficult conversation is because we *see it* as a conflict. When we perceive a difficult conversation as a confrontation, we are already mentally preparing for battle. If it's a battle, then of course we're either going to attack our enemy or defend ourselves.

Confrontation in its very essence is always something to be feared because it already implies that we are carrying weapons and armor into a difficult conversation; but if we *don't perceive* it as a confrontation, we won't perceive the person we're talking to as "the enemy."

There is no enemy, so there's no need for hostility. What there *is*, however, is a difficult situation or subject to be addressed. When you think about it, what we usually define as a confrontation is merely a very important *discussion* between parties to resolve an urgent matter.

Most of us are afraid of the consequences of how a difficult conversation will turn out. If we ask ourselves why we are afraid, our Surface-Layer Reasoning is that the other person might get angry or misunderstand us and things might get worse, so we don't want to risk it.

However, when we examine our Deeper-Layer Reasoning, we'll find that our fears manifest from our *own* expectations of what we *need* from the conversation. When we are amping ourselves up for a confrontation, we usually already feel strongly about the topic, so we actually have a need for the person to *understand us* and to *agree* with us.

This is the main problem with a difficult conversation—it's not the difficult subject that makes a conversation difficult, but the expectations, judgement, resentment, and ego that *bring hostility* to the table and make the conversation difficult.

Even people who love each other have simmering resentments and anger that comes from expectations, judgements, and hurt, and those are issues between people connected by bonds of the heart! It can be even more difficult at times with coworkers who are obligated to communicate with each other or strangers who have very different point of views. The hostility that comes along with our need to be right or for people to agree with us makes it hard for us not to react negatively when we are trying to communicate.

This is why it's so important for us to understand ourselves and *our objectives* before we go into a difficult conversation, because if we're not clear about why we're upset, ask—*Is it my expectations? Is it my ego?*—or not clear about our objectives—*Do I want the person to admit they're wrong, or do I want to solve this problem?*—then the way we communicate with someone will always be charged with expectations, judgement, resentment, and anger.

Often, we already feel wronged or hurt by the person, so when we try to talk to them and they react negatively, we are immediately triggered. We either feel attacked and back off due to fear or we feel so upset that we fight back even harder.

When we broach a difficult subject with someone, the objective needs to be to simply to *understand* that person; because if our objective is that we want the person to understand *us* and *our* logic, it *will* be a confrontation, since we will be ready to defend or attack the moment they don't understand us or disagree with us.

We *already know* it's a difficult subject going in, so *why* do we allow ourselves to get so triggered when it is difficult?

We *already know* that people are different, so *why* do we allow ourselves to get so triggered when people show us how different they are in terms of logic, principles, values, and beliefs?

We *already know* that the person whom we're talking to is likely to have a different opinion, so *why* do we allow ourselves to get so triggered when someone argues with us or defends themselves?

A difficult conversation is by its nature already difficult. But if we don't see it as a confrontation, we will be better equipped to respond in a manner that is more positive than negative, because in our minds, it will be just *two adults having a conversation.*

Sometimes, it is the *other person* who sees the difficult conversation as a confrontation, and they come in already in an aggressive mode and ready to attack or defend. Yet even then, it is up to us not to react to their reaction—even if the other person doesn't want to behave like an adult, that doesn't mean we cannot behave in an adult manner.

In life, it's important for us to choose a way of looking at difficult situations that helps us take positive action. For example, if someone were spreading rumors about you, you wouldn't need to fear approaching the person in question, because you wouldn't be *confronting* the person, your objective would merely be to find out the truth and understand what happened and why.

If we ever feel harassed in any way, it's absolutely necessary to *address the urgency and importance* of the matter. But seeing it as a "confrontation" just makes us more wary and fearful of doing something, which holds us back.

When we drop the idea of a confrontation, we drop our own hostility and expectations of how people "should respond" when entering a conversation about a difficult subject. That way, even if people don't respond positively, or if they become aggressive, *we* won't get so angry or so afraid that we can't take action to meet our own objectives when addressing the difficult situation at hand.

WHEN A PERSON TRIGGERS YOU, THANK THEM FOR TEACHING YOU SOMETHING ABOUT YOURSELF

<Acceptance>

When we have to communicate with someone we find difficult and challenging, it's natural for us to feel that *we* get along pretty well with everyone and that it's just this *one* particular person who is being contrary and troublesome.

With other people, there's no problem. With *you*, there's a problem. So it's easy to come to the conclusion that *you* are the problem.

This is why, even though we may understand the practices of self-awareness and emotional resilience, there is still so much resistance in letting go of our negative emotions toward a person we find difficult, because we're thinking, "Why should *I* have to work on it? Why not *you*?!"

This is why we often don't work on ourselves as much as is needed; we think we're actually quite good at being a happy person—we're having positive experiences with other people, so with the few people with whom we have negative experiences, it's easy to think that it's more *their* problem than ours.

It's very easy to self-reflect for a while, decide that we are not the problem, and then "let it go" in the sense of pushing the responsibility for practicing self-awareness and emotional resilience onto the other person. This is essentially us excusing ourselves from responsibility for our own reactions.

There are all sorts of people in this world. People can be entitled, ignorant, and rude, and they can contribute negatively to society.

It may indeed be absolutely true that the other person is less reasonable and more egotistical, yet if we find ourselves being triggered by this person, it is like having a sign light up that says, "Here, here! This is where I can work on myself!"

In fact, instead of being upset by people for triggering us, we should be thanking them for showing us where we should focus our inner work. Every single difficult person we come across is our teacher—they're showing us who we *don't want* to be, as well as giving us *an opportunity to practice* all the virtues that we say we would like to embody.

If no one challenges us, how can we grow as people? If we're never tested, how do we measure if we're actually progressing as human beings?

It's easy to be nice and rational when talking to someone else who's nice and rational, but how we do behave when we're faced with someone who irritates and angers us?

No matter how much we want to push the work onto someone else, every single one of our reactions is still our own responsibility. If we think, *"You should be more patient!"* it indicates that we are feeling impatience about others' impatience. If we find ourselves getting upset at someone's ego, it means that our own egos need attention, too.

As long as we think that *people* are the cause of our negative emotions and reactions, then we will never have a real need to figure out any other reason for the unhappiness that we feel. This is why even though our objective may be to grow as a person, if we're stuck in this pattern, we will see little or no progress; because if we pick and choose *when* to work on ourselves, then the reality is that we will get in very little practice.

Happiness is a practice. Regardless of whether *other* people are practicing it or not, *we* can always practice how to respond positively to challenging situations.

DO YOU RECOGNIZE THE VOICE OF YOUR EGO AND YOUR SELF-ESTEEM?

<Understanding>

No matter how different each individual is, we all share the commonality of having an ego as well as self-esteem. When our ego is larger than our self-esteem, we tend to be easily triggered by other people because we are not getting what we need to feel good about ourselves. When we understand this about ourselves, we understand this about other people.

Most of us don't think of ourselves as egotistical because we don't think we're arrogant. In fact, many of us think that we are considerate and humble, so it wouldn't even occur to us that our ego is in play when we are upset. This is why it's very important to understand the source of our reactions so that we can consciously feed our self-esteem and not accidentally feed our ego.

Often, our ego is so clever that it disguises itself as good intentions and positive standards, which is why it can be so hard to identify when our actions and reactions are ego-driven.

If we were to observe our conversations with our friends, we'd see that one of the reasons why we get along so well is because we share a similar worldview with them. This isn't to say that everyone agrees all the time, but that's why it can be fun to debate with a friend, because even if you end up agreeing to disagree, you still feel that fundamentally, the person is *more similar* than dissimilar to you.

This is because while good friends may have extremely diverse opinions and tastes, they rarely disagree with each other on the fundamentals of life. We get along extremely well with people who embrace values and beliefs similar to ours because as human beings, we are all incredibly drawn to people who reflect the different aspects of goodness we see in ourselves. We love being around people who are similar to us because they validate us, not in the sense that it makes us arrogant or vain, but rather providing the sort of validation that helps solidify and strengthen the very foundation of our identities.

When we interact with people who have beliefs, principles, and worldviews that are the opposite of ours, it can be really hard not to react negatively because it can feel like they are in opposition to the very *foundation of who we are*. When we interact with someone who represents the very opposite of what we believe in, it feels like they are objecting to our identities and who we are as people, which is why we take it so personally and find it so hard to remain calm. It's almost like their very existence is an insult to what we believe in, and we end up feeling that is the source of our frustration and negative reaction.

When we seek to understand, however, we can truly see that people are not objecting *to us*, they are simply being who they are in accordance with what is normal in their own reality. This is important for us to understand because when we find ourselves reacting negatively to people, it is a *signal* for us to feed our self-esteem so that we don't keep allowing our sense of our own identity depend on what other people say or do.

How well we understand our ego and our self-esteem drives how well how we *communicate* with people. If we cannot understand ourselves, we won't even be able to progress to talking about the *actual* situation with the person with whom we're trying to communicate. For example, if you and your colleague are having a disagreement during a meeting, you won't be able to have a conversation where you can explain your ideas in a way that is clear or can be understood by the person, because you will be too agitated by how *wrong* they are. This is what labeling someone as "difficult," "negative," or "stupid" does to us—our vibe and demeanor toward the person are already hostile and disbelieving, so much so that, even if we tell ourselves to be nice and to be patient, nothing works because our vibe has already sabotaged our efforts.

This is why we often feel like we are *already trying* to communicate with someone, and we come to the frustrating conclusion that *the person* is the problem—because we've tried so hard to be calm, understanding, and patient yet the person is not receptive at all!

We often don't realize that trying to be nice is actually futile if, when we enter the conversation, we already have a judgement of the person. The damage has already been done even before we start talking. All the niceties in the world cannot take away our belief about someone, because our belief about a person always manifests into a vibe that is clearer than any spoken language.

This goes for *every* person with whom we have difficulty communicating.

When it comes to family, we can often feel frustrated. For example, we can try so hard to be nice to our mother-in-law—even going as far as to please them—but she can remain as critical and as nasty as ever. Our frustration stems partly the fact that we've made so much effort with no results, partly from the disappointment that comes from the hope of making some headway and partly because of the injury to our pride that someone can dismiss us so easily.

Part of the reason why our pride can be injured is because, when we care about what someone thinks, it hurts when that person is showing an obvious dislike toward us. That's why it feels very personal. When our mother-in-law doesn't like us, it can feel like she is implying that we are "not good enough" and objecting to us as a human being, and that's why it matters so much.

All this misery builds up into a rage, and this rage causes us to be even more defensive and more bitter.

Usually, we'll be so upset we'll tell ourselves we don't care, but that doesn't actually take away the suffering we feel.

Most of us naturally want to improve a negative situation, or at the very least, we would much prefer to have good relations with people, especially the people we love. So even when we're not happy with someone, we usually try to make an effort by trying to think positively, making an effort to be kind, and maybe even going as far as to compromise to please them. Sometimes it works, but the majority of the time, we end up feeling increasingly frustrated, because despite all our efforts, the person doesn't respond as we think they should, and this makes us feel even more resentful of them.

When we break it down as to *why* we feel resentful, we can begin to explore the different ways in which we crave validation. By our nature, we human beings love the feeling of being liked; so by virtue of that, we experience huge discomfort around people we know don't approve of us or don't like us.

When someone responds positively, it indicates to us that we are doing something right. There is a subconscious sense of achievement or success when someone likes us. There is a feeling of satisfaction and reward when we have good chemistry with someone. Simply put, it feels good.

When someone *doesn't* respond positively, or at all, it doesn't feel good. When it doesn't feel good, it is very natural for us to put up a wall and react with anger to defend ourselves, as well as to default to blame so that we can feel better.

When it's someone else's fault, it's much easier to feel okay about it.

The reason I bring this up is not for us to feel bad or guilty, but to better understand ourselves and our triggers. Most of our suffering in our relationships with people comes from us needing the person to give us something back in return for all our effort—it's not that our efforts aren't genuine, it is that they are laced with expectations, judgements, and resentment. This is why even while we may put in a lot of effort to relate with someone, the person can still feel the lack of authenticity based on our reactions.

It is our ego's needs that lead to us reacting negatively when people don't like, acknowledge, or respect us; especially if we have *put in effort* to be likable. If we are not subconsciously seeking approval or validation, we won't be so bothered nor so negatively affected when people do not respond to us in the way that we hope.

This is the reason that, when it comes to difficult relationships, such as with a mother-in-law, we can think, *"Bah, I don't care what she thinks!"* yet still feel so affected every time we interact with her. We may truly not care what she thinks of us, but deep down inside, we feel extreme discomfort that she doesn't seem to see our good intentions.

A better way to approach this isn't to stop caring, but rather to feed our self-esteem so that we don't attach her words and actions to our sense of self. It's important to understand that when people are unkind, it stems from their own fears and insecurities and has nothing to do with us. It is only when we are acting from our ego that we seek validation, and that is when we will constantly tend to react negatively.

If we can understand ourselves, we will understand the needs and fears that manifest from our egos. Then, we can choose to not feed the ego and instead work on building stronger self-esteem.

When we are interacting with people with whom we disagree, the objective isn't to alter their personalities or change their minds, the objective is to change *how we feel* toward such people and situations as a whole so we don't continue to suffer.

When we observe what drives our actions and reactions, we will have powerful realizations about our relationships and interactions with people. It is powerful because once we see a perspective that can help us be happy, we cannot unsee it. When we understand something, we will never go back to how we used to see things. Once we understand the shape of our egos, we will begin to recognize when ego is driving our reactions, and this is extremely powerful in helping us remove the barriers to our happiness.

OFFENSE CAN CERTAINLY BE GIVEN, BUT IT DOESN'T HAVE TO BE TAKEN

<Understanding>

In a single day, how often and how easily can someone offend us?

When someone says something that upsets us, we have to ask ourselves if the reason we are taking it so personally is because we already have an insecurity or fear attached to the very thing the person is mentioning.

For example, if I am already insecure about my weight, I might be very insulted if you made a comment about how I look. If I am already afraid that I'm not good enough, then when you make a comment about my capabilities or intelligence, I might feel very criticized.

Most times, people are not trying to offend, insult, or criticize us, but we *receive* it as such. This is because the majority of the time, we see and hear through our own individual lens, which is colored by our own preconceived notions, history, experience, and conditioning. This means that when people say something to us, we are not just listening to their words, we are adding another layer of meaning onto it.

Once, when I was in Singapore to conduct a workshop, I was about to head out of my hotel when my mom—who was with me because she's my manager—asked, "Oh, I thought you were wearing the other dress?"

I immediately stopped and looked at her. "Why?" I asked, in a slight panic. "Is this not nice?"

"It's nice—I was just wondering why you wore this because you asked me to help iron the other dress."

Whew.

That small incident was significant for me, because I realized that I wasn't even hearing the *words* my mom was saying, I was hearing what I thought she was *implying*. This made me wonder— what else do I hear in a way that is different from someone's intended meaning?

Sometimes, people are not trying to offend us but we *feel* offended because we take it very personally, and this is why it's so important for us to understand ourselves.

If we are not aware of how our ego urges us to seek validation and respect externally, we can become very easily affected, to the point where we may easily be offended by every single person who disagrees with us—we'll see customer service personnel as "rude" when they don't bother smiling or speaking nicely, we'll see people who drive badly as "a**holes," and we won't realize it's our own *reaction* to them that is causing us to feel so upset.

Sometimes, people *do* have the intention to insult, offend, or criticize us. But here's the thing—offense can certainly be given, but it doesn't have to be *taken*.

If someone calls you a dog, all you have to do is to look behind you and check if you have a tail. If you don't have a tail, you're not a dog. If you're not what some people say you are, then why is it necessary to get upset over it?

Often, we react to what people say because we feel disrespected; but nobody can disrespect us if we respect ourselves. Our ego is wily enough to keep telling us that if people are insulting us or offending us and that we *should* feel insulted and offended. However, when we have healthy self-esteem, our self-esteem will tell us that nobody can insult or offend us if we choose not to attach our sense of identity to any other people's words and actions. Our self-esteem lets us know that if our foundation of identity is solid, nobody can shake it.

In life, not everyone will understand our intentions. Sometimes, we are hugely misunderstood, and we have to be okay with that, otherwise we will feel so wronged that we will not be able to let go of our negativity toward the person doing the misunderstanding. Sometimes, we are unfairly disliked, and we have to be okay with that, otherwise we will feel like "correcting" people and not be able to let go of our indignation.

This is why it's so important for us to build a healthy sense of self, because our ego will urge us to react and tell us things like, "*How dare they think badly of you!*" At the same time, our self-esteem will reassure us, "*It's okay for them to think what they do, as long as I am not choosing to let their opinions to make me feel bad about myself.*"

Which story are we telling ourselves?

To be human is to be vulnerable. We all have needs and fears which can very easily drive our reactions. This isn't a bad thing; it's just the way life works. This is why the most important relationship we can have is the relationship with ourselves, because if we don't understand our vulnerabilities and don't acknowledge what we fear, we won't want to let go of blame and anger as protective armor. We will suffer, not because of others, but because of what we ourselves cannot manage to release.

We can have a lot going for us, but if we're easily offended or upset by people, we will be in a constant state of unhappiness. Instead of putting so much energy into being upset over what people say about us, we can channel all that energy into the story *we tell ourselves*. If we have a strong foundation of self-love and self-acceptance, then it's very hard for people to put us down, even when they try to do so.

OTHER PEOPLE'S BAD BEHAVIOR DOES NOT JUSTIFY OUR OWN

<Awareness>

When people do something to us and we don't blame them, doesn't that mean we're letting them take advantage of us?

If you're nice even when people are nasty, doesn't that mean you're giving them permission to walk all over you?

When it comes to people treating us badly or taking advantage of us, much of the dilemma in our decision-making process seem to revolve around when we should be nice, when we should be less kind, and when we need to be more angry.

However, being kind and not angry are the practices we should adopt so that we can live life being the best version of ourselves— they are not traits that we put on and discard when necessary or convenient. Someone nice will always be nice, because that's *who they are.*

If someone told you that in order to get what you want, you had to be unkind and angry, what would you say?

Sometimes, we can be misled by our own ego into thinking that in order to solve a problem or achieve an objective, we *have* to be the worst version of ourselves. This is why, even though we may be sweet, wonderful people, we may feel completely righteous and justified in behaving in ways that are "not like ourselves." The ego tells us that we *should* stand up for ourselves and for others by saying or doing things aggressively.

In our minds, we believe that we are good people, and it's just that *in this situation* it is justified for us to behave in ways that we wouldn't "normally behave."

This is similar to saying, "I'm *normally* a nice person, it's just that your behavior left me no choice but to be mean," or, "I *have* to be nasty to you because you're such a terrible person."

It is the ego that deludes us into believing that we are nice people even when we are behaving like the worst version of ourselves, because only one's own ego can be so wily as to trick us into thinking that the only way to take action is through self-righteousness, even going as far as to justify our behavior as "necessary."

In reality, we are either nice or we are not nice. We either believe in letting go of negative emotions, or we believe in holding onto negative emotions. If we are "sometimes this" and "sometimes that," it means that we don't even know who we really are. If we don't know who we are, then we are always going to behave in accordance with how *other people behave,* and this is one of the key reasons why it's so hard for us to be fulfilled and happy: because our fulfilment and happiness depends so much on other people.

And the truth is, even if we decide that it's okay to unleash the worst version of ourselves upon someone, it doesn't mean that it's going to *help* us solve the problems at hand that we are facing. We have to remember that our real objective is to take the appropriate action to solve problems.

When we are interacting with someone we find difficult, we usually think that we can only choose from two options that lie at the opposite end of the spectrum—to be easily taken advantage of and nice, or to not be nice as a way to stand up for ourselves.

But those are not the only choices available to us. There is always a third option—we can be nice *and* stand up for ourselves. Being kind and being strong are not mutually exclusive. We don't need blame someone or get upset to stand up for ourselves, and being nice and kind does *not* mean that we are volunteering to let someone else take advantage of us. In fact, it's the opposite—it is when we don't allow people to change who we are or dictate the way we behave that others will never be able to take advantage of us.

WHEN PEOPLE TAKE ADVANTAGE OF US, WE DON'T NEED BLAME OR ANGER TO STAND UP FOR OURSELVES

<Understanding>

One night over dinner, my mom casually said to the family, "So... I'm not sure I did the right thing, but I gave the washing machine repairman RM800 (the equivalent of 200 US dollars) in cash in advance to buy spare parts to repair my washing machine and dryer."

She went on to tell us that it was only after he left that it occurred to her that it might be a risk to give money to a freelance repairman, as there was less accountability than with a company.

However, this guy, Harry, was someone who had been to my mom's house as well as my house to repair our machines, since he used to work for the company where we'd bought our washing machines and dryers. So he wasn't a total stranger, and after he left his job with the company, he continued to repair our machines on a freelance basis with no problem.

In any case, my mom reasoned, "It makes sense that I had to give him money up front, otherwise he wouldn't have the money to buy the parts needed to repair my washing machine and dryer."

Harry wasn't well off, so it did make sense. Besides, my mom said she trusted him as he'd done jobs at the house before.

However, right after he left with the money, my mom did have a niggling feeling that maybe she should have asked Harry for a copy of his identification for insurance purposes. The only thing she had was his full name, mobile number, and his bank account number, which wasn't much to work with should he choose not to honor their deal.

And guess what? That was exactly what happened! Harry did not fulfil his promise to fix the machine, instead giving the excuse that the spare parts were not available each time my mom called. After close to a month of the same excuses, my mom decided to cancel the arrangement with Harry, at which time he agreed to refund her money. She went on to get her machines repaired by a reputable company.

Harry's promise to refund my mom's money, however, went unhonored. Over the course of the next few months, my mom continued to text him and he again promised to refund the money, but to no effect. This song-and-dance cycle went on for five whole months, at which point it was crystal clear that he had no real intention of paying her back.

The strange thing was that Harry would still reply to messages my mom left him, even going as far as to give a time and date when he said he would transfer the money to her bank account; but the day would come and go without any refund payment.

Of course, my mom was understandably upset that he would do such a thing. I think she was more upset at the fact that he would cheat a sixty-one-year-old woman than about the money itself!

My mom wasn't so much angry at him as she was *disappointed* in him. All her texts to him were stern and serious but never angry. She even congratulated him on his marriage when he told her he would pay her back after the wedding because he needed the money. But of course, after the wedding, there was still no money.

She would show me all his texts with unbelievable excuses, and we would exclaim over how terrible it was, but she wasn't filled with frustration or anger. What had happened had already happened. My mom told me that being angry with him wouldn't make him pay her back, and being frustrated would just ruin her own day.

Emotionally, she had already let go.

My mom is retired and is very careful with how she spends her money, but she said, "If I don't get my money back, I'll think of it as a donation. For someone to cheat you of your money, they would have to be in desperate need of it."

Letting it go emotionally allowed her to accept the situation without it involving the suffering of anger toward him or regret over her decision to trust him. Since this situation had already occurred, she had two choices: to pursue it, or to not pursue it.

In her case, she decided to pursue it. She first obtained his identification information by looking through the security records at the guardhouse at her residence, where all visitors, including Harry, had to sign in with their personal details before proceeding into the housing area. Then, my mom proceeded to make a report at the police station and finally followed it up with a tribunal hearing.

It could be seen as going to too much trouble with no guarantee that it would result in her getting her money back, but my mom's reasoning for pursuing the case was that if she didn't take action, Harry would think that it's perfectly okay to cheat people and might continue doing it to others.

"If I let him get away with this, I'm not doing him any favors. My objective is not to punish him, but to help him learn that there are consequences to what he's doing," she told me. She focused on her two objectives—to not suffer, and to help him learn that there are consequences to his actions.

And lo and behold, just before the tribunal hearing, Harry paid my mom back!

From the wording of his messages and the way he challenged my mom to show him proof that she had gone to the police, I think that he didn't believe that my mom would go that far. But when he received the summons to appear for a hearing at the tribunal, he finally realized that he might be facing some serious charges in court.

There's no guarantee that he won't ever do this to other people in the future, but I'm pretty sure he now understands that it's not so easy to get away with it, and that might help him think twice.

I accompanied her both to the police station and to the tribunal and saw firsthand all that unfolded. Harry had clearly taken advantage of my mom, yet she was never the victim.

Firstly, my mom wasn't a victim because she didn't allow this incident to change her into a less trusting person—she likes the fact that she's open and not suspicious of people, because it makes the majority of her interactions and relationships so much more joyful. She wasn't nasty to Harry because she isn't a nasty person, and to allow Harry to change that about her would be illogical.

Instead of letting this experience make her more jaded, more wary, more suspicious, and generally more unhappy, my mom has simply chosen to see this as an experience that has given her valuable information as to how people can behave. With this experience and information, she will be better informed in the future on what cautionary measures to take in similar situations.

Secondly, my mom wasn't a victim because she didn't allow someone else's actions to make her feel bad. It was obvious that Harry had cheated her, yet she was able to remain calm because she understood that the situation has already unfolded—it had already happened, so she accepted it. Being angry wouldn't have helped change what had happened and would only have made her feel worse.

Lastly, my mom wasn't a victim because instead of beating herself up for her mistake, she took action. She knew that what Harry had done was not right. So regardless of what her efforts might yield, she went through the legal process to show him that there were consequences to his actions.

To observe all of this unfolding was interesting, because my mom once again showed me that we don't have to be "mean" in order to stand up for ourselves.

Often, it is blame and anger that make us victims, because feelings of anger and righteousness make us *feel* as if we have taken action, but in fact, we may not have *actually taken action*. If we were in my mom's shoes, some of us might *not* have pursued the case to the police or the tribunal, because that took a lot of effort. But would we have been mad as hell? Very likely!

This means that we would have "let go" and "held on" to the wrong thing, in the sense that we would have held on to anger (which doesn't help us) and let go of taking the necessary action to address or solve the situation (which possibly can help us).

Often, we feel like victims because someone has done something to us. However, while it is true that one can be a victim to someone's actions, we don't have to be victimized if we always address the situation or solve the problem in the way that causes us the least suffering.

The thing is, it always takes more effort to figure out how to solve a problem than it does to be angry. Even when it's something small—like when someone is rude to us—it is easier to just get angry than to approach the person to tell them why their behavior was unacceptable. So when it's something bigger—like we're feeling like someone has taken advantage of us, it's also easier to blame someone and get angry than to actually address the situation in order to change it.

All of us have boundaries and definitions of what we find unacceptable when it comes to our interactions and relationships with people, and we can and must stand up for ourselves. However, being effective is not about being "unkind," but about solving problems without allowing the situation to turn you into someone you're not proud to be. We don't need anger to convey the boundaries of what is unacceptable.

We can always take the necessary action to resolve something without the emotional baggage and suffering that come with anger and blame. However, if we choose not to take action, it is to our own benefit to make the conscious choice to also let go of our negative emotions toward the person or incident.

It helps to remember that choosing to let go of emotional suffering is already one form of positive action.

CHAPTER FOUR

Letting Go of Anger and What Doesn't Serve Us

PEOPLE DON'T "DO" THINGS TO US, THEY DO THINGS TO THEMSELVES

<Understanding>

When we are kids, we have little or no idea about the concept of taking responsibility for our own happiness, so whenever something undesirable happens, it's natural that we react according to what people have "done to us."

Now that we are adults, we have the capacity to understand that people don't "do" things to us—they just do what is characteristic for them to do. If it is characteristic of someone to lose their temper, they'll do it. If it's characteristic of them to bully others or to treat people with disrespect or disregard, they'll do that.

People can indeed behave badly, but they're not doing it *to* us, it's just that sometimes we happen to be unfortunate enough to experience or witness these characteristics of theirs. Sometimes we witness these traits in strangers or work colleagues, and sometimes we have family members, lovers, or friends who have negative characteristics, and that's why they seem to always be doing things that hurt us.

As adults, we have the ability to see that every hurtful thing that people do is a reflection of their own pain. Every judgement, blame, resentment, and anger that people have toward others is a reflection of how they feel about *themselves*. This means that even if someone has ill intent toward us, it is because of *their own* insecurities and issues, which manifest in their inability to love and to be kind.

Understanding this is so important for our happiness, because if we hold on to blame and anger, we are not standing up for ourselves—we are giving these same people power over our emotional wellbeing.

People can create situations that cause us a great deal of inconvenience or even pain. This is why it is so important to understand that they are not doing anything *to us*. This one thought—that "someone did something to me"—renders us immediately powerless.

We empower ourselves by understanding that even though it *feels* personal, it is *not* personal. When we don't take it personally, it means that we are not allowing *their* issues to become *our* issues. We are not allowing *their* unhappiness to become *our* unhappiness.

While we may at times be victims of others' actions, we won't have let them victimize us if we don't attach our sense of identity and self-worth to their actions. People may be able to affect our lives through the hurt, problems, and challenges they create, but they cannot make us less *significant* as human beings if we understand that their actions have never been about us.

If someone we love betrays us, it can feel very much like they did something terrible to us. That could be our belief. Or alternatively, our belief could be they did something terrible, full stop. The person didn't do anything *to* us, they made a decision in their own life that has impacted us. When people leave us, it doesn't mean they've discarded us. Nobody can treat us like garbage if we understand that their actions are not a reflection of us—their actions are a reflection of them.

We always have to take action to address what has happened, but we don't have to attribute blame to others for ruining our lives, because we understand that our lives are not ruined. Nobody should hold that kind of power over our quality of life and our happiness, so we don't have to give our power away by holding onto blame and anger for what people have "done to us."

This chapter is dedicated to how we can let go of what doesn't serve us, and more importantly, *why* it benefits our happiness to let go.

LETTING GO IS NEVER FOR THE PERSON WHO WRONGED US—IT'S FOR OURSELVES

<Acceptance>

One of the biggest factors holding us back from letting go is the belief that if we forgive people who hurt us, we are giving them permission to hurt us, or feel that we have to welcome them back into our lives.

Forgiving someone is not saying, "Please come back into my life," and it's definitely *not* saying, "I'm allowing you to do that to me again."

Forgiveness and letting go of hate are by no means about being a victim or being passive. Forgiving others is definitely not about us being submissive or giving the signal that it's okay for people to take advantage of us. When someone has hurt you and you forgive them, it does not automatically imply that you condone their actions or that you're letting them off easy.

Forgiveness and letting go are important because of just one thing—and that is our happiness and peace of mind. It's important for us to exit any interaction that is toxic, not just physically, but mentally and emotionally, too; and that means we don't volunteer to carry around hate or any emotion that causes us suffering.

Wishing someone ill, hoping that they will get what's coming to them, wanting them to suffer because of what they did—we believe that thinking this way will make us feel better and lighter, but often we end up feeling worse and heavier, weighed down by the bitterness in our hearts.

When we don't forgive someone, we think that we are making the person suffer and that they will continue to feel bad all the way to their grave—but it is not possible to impose conscience on another person. When you don't forgive, it just means that you are the only one who still cares.

So if someone has done something to you that is unforgivable, there is only one thing to do: forgive them.

Forgiveness is the key to truly ending our own suffering.

If you've already suffered once because of someone else's actions, not forgiving them is suffering twice, or a million times; because even if you don't see the person anymore, even if time has passed, you'll still feel the pain again each and every time you think of the person or the incident.

If someone has left physical scars on you, don't allow them to leave emotional scars too.

When someone has wronged you, think of how they must be suffering to say and do those things. Only someone truly unhappy would behave that way toward another human being. Every hurt they inflict, every temper tantrum they throw, and every abuse they dish out—each is caused by their own inability to be happy.

When we really look deep within ourselves, we may find that a big part of the reason why we don't want to forgive is because forgiveness feels too much like signifying that what someone did to us doesn't matter, when in fact it matters so darn much.

And if it doesn't matter, then it signifies that we don't matter.

Often, it's not because we don't want to let go, but we don't want what letting go might symbolize—that we've lost, that we're not significant, that we don't matter.

This is where the only thing that can ease our pain is to truly be able to see that letting go is about being significant; it's about living in such a way that nothing that anybody does to us can make us feel small. Letting go is a way of saying "I haven't lost, because you can't take my quality of life away from me." Letting go is the biggest and most important way of proclaiming to ourselves that we matter.

To forgive is not to excuse someone for what they did. We forgive to let go.

There is a saying in Mandarin, "放开别人是放过自己," that translates into, "We forgive others to free ourselves."

The best thing we can possibly do for our own lives is to free ourselves from the people who have hurt us. We can determine to live a happy life and not be consumed by toxicity, because at the end of the day, nobody can take the value of our lives away from us. If someone has caused us pain, we can choose not to let them cause us suffering by letting go of blame or anger.

Letting go is never for the people who've wronged us, it's for ourselves and our own happiness.

DON'T LET YOUR PAIN OF THE PAST STOP YOU FROM FULLY LIVING IN THE PRESENT

<Acceptance>

When my dad told my mom that he had met someone else and wanted to be with her, my mom didn't yell or object. She looked at him and quietly said, "Okay."

"Is that all you have to say?" he asked, surprised.

"Well, you've already decided. What else would you want me to say?"

This isn't to say that my mom wasn't shocked, but even with all the emotions she felt—betrayal, hurt, letdown, disappointment— her reaction wasn't that it was *unfair*. The thought never crossed her mind, because she didn't think that my dad was doing anything "to her." She understood that he was behaving in a way that was a reflection of his own state of mind.

She was upset, but she didn't stay upset because she didn't hold on to anger. This absence of anger would be hard for many people to comprehend, because how can a person feel betrayed yet not be angry?

For my mom, it was possible, because she didn't blame my dad. Without blame, there is often very little anger, which means that there is also very little standing in the way of accepting "what is."

In life, there is no other truth other than "what is"—what is happening, is what is happening. Wishing things were different or being upset that things aren't different doesn't change your reality. This doesn't mean we cannot feel upset, but it does mean that we can acknowledge how we feel with acceptance.

The acceptance of "what is" is not defeat, it is empowerment. This is because accepting "what is" helps us to be truly present instead of reliving the past or projecting into the future. Our suffering comes from our thoughts about how the past could have been different and our thoughts of how we wish for the future to be; yet in life, only the *present* exists. Being absolutely present in our lives is where we are at absolute peace—not wishing that the past was different or worrying about the future.

Since she is human, my mother has all the emotions that we human beings feel. The thing that I've always found extremely unique about my mom is the innate peace she has with who she is as a person. In her life, she has had some people treat her badly and take advantage of her, yet my mom has never *reacted* badly, because there is always a level of self-respect and self-love that is present—my mom doesn't attach her sense of who she is as a person to other people's actions, because she already feels valued as a person.

Her acceptance of herself means that she needs very little external validation—her self-esteem has always been bigger than her ego— and therefore she can always understand that people are not doing anything "to her" but merely behaving according to *their own* needs and fears. So whenever someone's actions affect her, she doesn't let them take away the value she has placed upon her own life. This is the main reason why my mom can always respond to difficult situations in a way that focuses on her objective—to not suffer and to be happy. Nobody can take her happiness away from her because she doesn't give her power away to people or things.

Accepting "what is" can *feel* like the opposite of standing up for ourselves—it would be very easy to mistake my mom's acceptance for not standing up for herself in the situation described above. However, as can be seen in the stories in this book, my mom has always been able to take the necessary actions to do what she believes is right without the need for anger and blame.

This was how my mom raised me and my brother, too. She has never once blamed us for what we did wrong, she simply took the necessary actions to talk to us to show us and guide us to how we can do right. Instead of us thinking that she was a pushover or easy to bully, her lack of anger and blame made us respect her, because she was always calm enough to firmly explain the error of our ways to us without making us feel guilty.

While I was growing up with my mom, this was always something interesting for me to observe—my mom feels all the emotions other people feel, yet she has always been able to act and not react because she doesn't give her power away. To her, no matter what people do that affects her, letting them dictate her happiness and her actions would be akin to being a victim, and my mom would never want that.

Blame is a huge part of what makes us miserable. When we think, "It's his/her fault!" it is because we want some kind of justification or closure. We want the offending person to feel bad, but it is unlikely that they'll feel repentant or remorseful. We want that person to take responsibility, but it is unlikely they'll do anything that will give us what we seek—people don't magically feel compelled to change just because we become angry and blame them.

Blaming someone doesn't correct their wrongs or make things right, but it definitely does give us more unhappiness. How are we to be happy when blame brings out the worst in us? When we blame people, we experience a series of negative emotions and reactions—we want blood, punishment, revenge; we want the person shamed and embarrassed.

The worst part is that blame makes us feel justified in feeling and behaving negatively, almost as if someone else's bad behavior has given us permission to be the worst version of ourselves. That's what the blame-mindset does to us—it turns us vindictive and equally deserving of blame as they are.

Other people can create situations that affect our happiness, but it is our own worldview that makes us miserable. If our worldview is that it's "right" and "just" to blame someone because it is their fault, that is as good as putting our happiness in the hands of that person, because we are stuck in reacting to what another person is doing to us.

This is a huge reason why we can so easily be unhappy with life—
without knowing it, we have time and again put our happiness
at the mercy of people and circumstances. In that mindset, the
minute something goes wrong, we will always be in the habit of
looking outwards for solutions to our misery instead of looking
inwards for how to be happy.

Blame makes it harder to take positive action because when we're
in this state of mind, we are too focused on anger. This is where
it becomes easy to lose sight of our objective of living a quality
and happy life. When blame is absent, all we need to focus on is
our approach for the best outcome: "An undesirable situation has
already occurred. It's not my fault that it happened, but it's my
responsibility to take care of myself. Now, what can I do so that I
don't suffer?"

This means we don't allow our pain of the past to stop us from
fully living in the present. We are making a conscious decision to
move toward and improve our future instead of getting stuck in
the past because we can't let go.

SATISFACTION ONLY DISGUISES ITSELF AS HAPPINESS

<Understanding>

Not a single person we speak to will say, "I don't want to be free from the pain of my past."

However, when someone has hurt us or caused us harm, we also don't want to let go, because "What about justice?!"

"Fulfilment of vengeance, that's very important," a friend said to me when I brought this up; "If someone does something to you, you feel like you want them to pay."

This is a feeling I can definitely relate to. In fact, I think that this is something almost every human being can relate to as an experience—how can we let people "get away" after they've caused irreparable damage to our lives?

So here we are—we want to be free from pain, but we don't want to let go because we believe that we must get even somehow. When you think about it, someone may have caused us pain in the past, but it is *this dilemma* that is causing us to suffer *in the present*.

I used to wholeheartedly believe in a black-and-white interpretation of the world. If you've read chapter two's "It's not personal, even when it feels personal," you know that initially I was a proponent of the death penalty, and that it was only later in life that I started to question my own beliefs about fairness and justice.

When I started to ask myself what objectives I hoped to accomplish with my insistence on getting even, the answer was always that my objectives were to achieve fairness and justice. I was extremely comfortable with the thought of punishing someone or making them suffer for what they'd done. Perhaps I even relished the idea of someone getting what was coming to them.

I had to ask myself: "This *desire* for justice and vengeance, where is it coming from?"

Our reaction of wanting to hurt another human being is driven by an animal instinct to protect ourselves and the people we love. However, when we return to rationality, we'll see that if something awful has already happened, it has already happened. No matter how much pain we inflict upon the perpetrator, it does *nothing* to erase the facts. This isn't about being matter-of-fact or making light of something extremely important—it is about understanding that all the hatred, anger, and retribution in the world cannot take away what has happened.

When something has already happened, the *most important thing* to determine is "What actions can I take from here that will give me the closure I need, that'll make sure I'm safe, and that'll help me live my life in a way that brings joy and happiness?"

If someone committed murder, I would definitely want them to be removed from society where they could not hurt or harm anyone again.

If someone has hurt me or the people I love, I would take action by determining how to best make sure they wouldn't be able to do it again.

There is a difference between *taking action* and *seeking justice.* We can take action without burning anger that traps us into suffering.

One of the main reasons why we seek vengeance is because we want closure. Yet even when we have inflicted punishment and pain on someone who has hurt us, it will still be very hard to get the closure we need if we cannot let go of anger and blame.

The idea that other people can give us closure only makes us more powerless—why give away more power to people who have already taken something away from us? Just as nobody can give us happiness, nobody can give us closure no matter how desperately we seek it, because closure is something that we can only give to ourselves.

We will find the closure we seek not from the person who caused us pain, but from understanding and having compassion for our own pain and choosing to let go of our suffering by releasing our anger, hatred, and thirst for vengeance.

The term *thirst for vengeance* already indicates that we can drink and drink and still be thirsty for more. People may have hurt us, but sometimes, we're not even aware that it is us who continue to hurt ourselves. Anger and blame make us so blind we often cannot see the forest for the trees.

This idea that vengeance can give us closure, or that justice needs to be something like, "If you made me suffer, you must suffer one hundred times my pain" is hugely perpetuated by the movies we watch. When we watch a movie where it's very clear who the villain is, we feel this absolute sense of satisfaction when the bad guys "get what's coming to them." This sense of justice is what we viewers need to feel—if the bad guy doesn't die or suffer horribly by the end of the movie, we'll feel rather cheated! That wasn't a good movie!

Revenge sounds really good, but in real life, someone else's suffering doesn't give us peace. The idea of getting even does give us *huge satisfaction,* and that is a very sad thing indeed—that we need to partake in someone else's suffering just so we're not alone in our own.

Tracking down this train of thought made me aware of something about myself—I *really like* the feeling of satisfaction. Acknowledging this is interesting, because it makes me check myself and helps me be more aware when I am seeking satisfaction through righteous anger and might be sabotaging my own happiness. It's very human of us to seek some form of satisfaction, especially when it comes to seeing the people who have hurt us—or even the people we don't like—get what we think they deserve.

Understanding this about myself made me question everything. What, actually, do people deserve? Do they deserve punishment? Do they deserve death?

And ultimately, *why does it matter to us what other people deserve?*

If we have to focus even an *ounce* of our energy on something, we should be focusing on what *we deserve*—we deserve to live our lives in the best way we possibly can, through all the challenges, hurt, and pain that inevitably come our way.

In the same way that nobody else can give us closure, nobody can give us what we deserve—because nobody can live our lives for us.

It wasn't until I started examining this from all angles that I realized fairness and justice weren't actually my *real* objectives— that sense of satisfaction does feel good, but what's my actual objective in life?

When I think that something is not right, my objective is to take action to address the situation and to bring it to a better place. So the question is, what do I mean by a "better place"? Better for my satisfaction? Or better for my happiness?

My ego—the part of me that seeks outside significance and validation—pushes for satisfaction.

My self-esteem—the part of me that tells me I am already significant and always worthy—reminds me that my happiness is something nothing and no one can take away from me.

Do I want to feed my ego? Or do I want to grow my self-esteem? Our ego and our self-esteem live side by side, as two halves of something that make a whole. If we choose to feed the ego, our self-esteem naturally shrinks to make space—this is why in life, we can grow in satisfaction but still feel extremely unfulfilled.

If we choose to feed our self-esteem, the ego becomes smaller to pave the way for a stronger sense of self—this is why some people are able to live a very fulfilled life even after experiencing incredibly painful or heartbreaking events. A strong self-esteem means that we believe in our own worth and the value of our life enough to not give our happiness away to circumstances and people.

Satisfaction is *not happiness*, and if we're not aware, it's very easy to confuse the two.

My *real* objective, I realized, is not to seek ego satisfaction through anger or to be tricked into thinking I can get closure through revenge. My real objective in life is to live each day with peace and happiness.

To achieve this objective, it means that when someone has hurt or harmed me, I *cannot let the person victimize me further by holding onto righteous anger and my need for revenge.*

Because doing that would mean having to live in the past, and that would rob me of my freedom in the present.

We cannot have ice in our veins and hate in our hearts yet want to live with peace and love. This is why we don't forgive for the sake of others, but for ourselves. It's in our own self-interest not to hold ourselves back by holding on to anger, hatred, and blame. If we really want revenge, then we can take it by living our best life.

TAKE THE THORN FROM
YOUR HEART AND
THROW IT AWAY

<Acceptance>

When I became old enough to be bothered by things and people, my mom would say to me, "Girl, take the thorn from your heart and throw it away."

Every time she said it, she would use the movement of her hand to mimic removing an imaginary thorn from her heart and flinging it far away.

She'd say, "When you can't let go, you're not hurting the other person, you're hurting yourself, because you'll feel the thorn stabbing your heart again and again."

I could see the sense in what she was saying, but it wasn't until I had to truly put it into practice that I understood exactly what she meant. Once when I had just started my career, there was an incident at work—to my absolute dismay, I discovered that a colleague was being vindictive and was spreading rumors about me in a blog post she had written before she even met me. I felt truly betrayed when I discovered that, as I had considered her a friend.

It was a double betrayal, because she was also the public relations personnel for the company—I was a new talent for the television network where we were both employed, and it was her job to secure publicity for me and the show. I felt stabbed in the back both personally and professionally.

Because it was a serious work issue, we were both called into meetings with her boss and my producers to address it. She apologized profusely and gave assurances that she would never do anything like that in the future. True to her word, she never again did anything remotely negative toward me.

Although I didn't want to allow her actions to affect me emotionally, I couldn't fully let it go. I felt like everyone should know what kind of person she was, and it irked me to no end that I had friends who thought she was a wonderful person. I've always felt the urge since then to *tell* people what she did; but after I did that once or twice, I realized that I was coming across as very bitter and negative, and that wasn't the sort of person I wanted to be.

It's funny how when someone has done something to us, we want to tell the world about their "true nature," which is ironic, because the desire to do that comes from our need for significance, which says a lot about our own nature.

I wouldn't admit it (even to myself) back then, but I wanted some sort of justice. My mom reminded me that as long as I didn't remove that thorn from my heart, I was going to be uncomfortable and disturbed every time I saw this co-worker in person or even heard her name mentioned.

My mom was right. That was when I learned that removing the thorn from my heart wasn't a one-time thing—it was a *practice*.

At times I was sure that I'd plucked the thorn out and thrown it away, but then when I saw this woman again, I would still feel negatively toward her. Those were the moments where I had to be incredibly honest with myself: Why am I reacting this way? What does my ego need? Is it actually helping me, or is it making me feel worse?

We can *say* that we're not angry or upset, yet we can't lie to ourselves when we feel an emotional charge. Even our bodies react to it—our hearts beat faster, and we're more agitated.

I also realized that it's *not about the other person*. This woman's reputation and credibility was called into question by her own boss, which I have to say did give me a sense of satisfaction at the time. However, I realized that the quantity of another person's pain does not translate into our having the ability to let go—the thorn can still be as deeply imbedded in our hearts as ever.

This is why even when criminals are put away, even when the people who hurt us suffer, we still cannot live our lives freely and joyously.

The practice of releasing these feelings starts with a genuine desire to let go. We can think we've let go when we've settled the issue, but we also need to let go *emotionally*. It's a process of feeling those thorny sensations and being willing to acknowledge that our desire to seek retribution comes from our need for validation or significance.

Anger is interesting, because every time we experience the emotion, we're also discovering something about ourselves. We often think that people cause us to be angry, but anger is our *own emotion*. At its source, anger doesn't come from others, it comes from deep within us.

Only we can take the thorn from our hearts and throw it away.

As for my friend, I saw her again years later at a mutual friend's wedding, and we all went out for supper together. That night, we sat next to each other and caught up, and I had such a great time. I genuinely enjoyed talking to her and listening to her stories. It felt amazing, and it was such a relief to know that the thorn has well and truly been taken out and thrown away!

RIGHTEOUS ANGER IS NOT SELF-PRESERVATION, IT'S SELF-SABOTAGE

<Understanding>

One of the main reasons we find it so hard to let go of anger and blame is because it can feel like doing so goes against our instincts of self-preservation and standing up for what's right.

Most of us don't particularly like feeling anger, but we do think, "Hey, sometimes you have to be angry to draw the line and show someone what is unacceptable."

Righteous anger happens when we feel upset and we think that we have a *right* to be upset. It is the kind of anger that we feel *needs* to be there—it makes us feel like we are correcting a wrong, when in actual fact, we are *perpetuating* a wrong.

The biggest irony of righteous anger is that we truly believe that we are *virtuous* for feeling angry, because we feel like we're standing up for something. We all have such strong beliefs, values, and principles that it's actually quite difficult *not* to feel righteous when it comes to how "good" we feel we are. Most of us know that we're not perfect, but we are proud of the guiding principles by which we live. When someone behaves in a way that is the opposite of how we would behave, there is a strange sense of righteous satisfaction in feeling angry because our show of anger is a way to highlight how *we are better than that*.

When we feel righteously angry, we're not in fact consciously thinking, "Aha! It's because I'm better!" We genuinely believe that we are standing up for what's right. But when we examine our Deeper-Layer Reasoning, we might find that the reason it feels so satisfying to be angry is because the angrier we get, the more it validates how good a person we are.

This is why without even being aware of it, we can very easily be a member of the *Hate the Haters Club*. This is where we find ourselves imposing our standards on people and judging them based on what we would or wouldn't do, and then feeling incredibly justified in showing our anger and hatred toward them.

This is why righteous anger is incredibly ironic—it is only in our quest to do good that we start behaving in a manner that is exactly like what we say we hate!

If we are really better than the people whose actions we condemn, then it means that we are *wiser*, and that wisdom would be helping us to be *less* judgmental, rather than *more* judgmental.

Logically, no matter how ignorant, obnoxious, inconsiderate, or inhumane we think someone is, wishing them ill just does not reflect how we are any better. If we see someone abusing a dog, we get angry because we believe that since that is a very unkind act, it is therefore *right* to be angry. According to this belief, getting angry signifies that *we* think we are kind, and that we're not "that sort of person."

However, *if we are indeed kind*, we wouldn't get so angry that we wish the abuser all kinds of slow, painful torture and death; because that is surely not the best way to show by example what kindness is.

We may not be an abuser, but in hating an abuser, we too are exhibiting abusive behavior toward that person. Righteous anger can lead us to exhibit *the same behavior* we say we want to eliminate.

This is why the concepts of just retribution and revenge sound very good in theory, but when we seek to implement them, we become the *very thing* we do not believe in—we become the very people we hate.

Righteous anger is such a formidable foe—it makes us think we're fighting for what's right when we're actually contributing more to what's *wrong*. It sabotages us.

Even when we are aware of this, we may still feel justified in harboring anger at someone, because we feel that, unlike ourselves, *they deserve it.* In fact, if we don't get angry, we feel it would be as if we're condoning their actions! We have to take a stand against what we believe is wrong, don't we?

Indeed, it is extremely helpful to do something about what we strongly believe is not right—action has to be taken. However, anger only *feels* like an action; but anger is merely an emotion. We *feel* like we're doing something, but in truth we're not creating any real change. This is where righteous anger sabotages us yet again!

Being righteously angry makes us feel like we are doing something, yet often, we are *only angry.* When you really think about it, anger only fuels our sense of ego satisfaction; it doesn't mean we are addressing the problem. This is why there is a huge difference between *right* and being *self-righteous.* When we think we are right, there is no need for anger—we can just take action to right the wrong.

"Take action?" a viewer commented when I was talking about righteous anger over a live video broadcast online. "Wow! I am so motivated to pour a can of paint on the person's car!"

I laughed out loud, because the visual of pouring paint over a person's car was the perfect imagery of what the satisfaction of revenge would feel like. How many times have we *entertained the thought* of doing something horrendous to someone to *make them pay* for the problems they've caused us?

The funny thing is, when we cause people suffering this way, we can *still feel like we're good people!* When we take revenge, we can still *believe* that we're *better* than the person upon whom we're exacting revenge!

Righteous anger can make us slightly delusional as to what our true nature is. It helps us justify our weaknesses, so we then have no reason to work on them. If everyone else is the problem, then I have no reason to work on myself, so my growth as a person will be very minimal, which means that I am a lot less wise than I fancy myself to be.

Swearing at someone we think is rude *is* an action, but we can't delude ourselves into thinking that we are "standing up for what's right" when in truth, we are putting more rudeness into the world.

When we see something that is not right in this world, we can take *positive* action. We have core values that we think are good, so we can *spread them* by *practicing* our core values in our daily lives.

Complaining, swearing, judging, and condemning people are not actions that will spread our good values, but signs that we feel the need to put other people down to highlight how "good" we are.

If we truly have better principles, beliefs, and values—if we truly are wiser—then it means we have more capacity for wisdom and understanding, which implies that we know how to solve problems by taking *positive actions* without bringing anger and hatred into the equation.

We don't suffer when we adhere to our own core values and codes of conduct. We suffer when we project our core values onto other people and judge them based on our them. There is no such thing as "right anger," because anger is anger—nobody is at peace when they're angry. Even when we are indignantly right and righteously angry, we will continue to be negatively affected.

In life, we can only be the change we want to see in the world. We can always fight for the greater good by *being* the greater good— not by hating the haters.

An eye for an eye simply results in two half-blind people—we call it justice, but really it's just making the whole world blind. We can choose to further perpetuate darkness and negativity by returning the hate that we see, or we can choose otherwise. We have to be careful not to turn into the very people we say we dislike. Remember that righteous anger only *disguises* itself as a powerful friend, when in reality it is a most powerful foe.

If we find ourselves constantly unhappy and unable to let go of what doesn't serve us, we have to ask ourselves if it's because deep down inside, we *don't want* to let go.

We want to be happy, but we don't *want* to change, because we feel it's not fair.

We want to be happy, but we don't *want* to accept things as they are, because we feel we are right.

We want to be happy, but we don't *want* to let go, because it feels like justice to hold on.

Most of us want to know *how* to let go. We want to jump ahead to being able to immediately let go of what doesn't serve us, but first we have to be able to *recognize* what doesn't serve us.

It is only when we are able to recognize how toxic righteous anger is that we will truly *want* to let go.

DO WE SEEK TO EMPOWER OURSELVES OR TO CONTROL OTHERS?

<Understanding>

Besides the feeling of righteousness, one of the biggest reasons why we don't want to let go of anger is because anger makes us feel we're in control—it feels like we're empowering ourselves.

When we are trying to get some kind of control over how people are treating us, anger is the most immediate and direct way to show someone that "You're not the boss of me" or "I'm not afraid of you."

This is what makes anger such an interesting emotion, because even though we often don't like ourselves when we're angry, being angry also feels empowering because we feel we're standing up for ourselves and not letting people push us around.

This is why anger isn't just satisfying, it can also be oddly comforting, because it makes us feel stronger. But this sense of power and strength is all an illusion. Instead of *giving us* power, anger *robs* us of power. We only *think* we're in control.

All we have to do to see the truth of this is to reflect on how we've behaved when we were consumed by anger. If we could look back at a video recording of what we said or how we behaved when we were angry, we might say, "I don't recognize myself."

This illustrates how although anger gives the illusion of strength and power, it is actually temporary insanity—we're not ourselves when we're angry, and the worst thing is, we *cannot see it* through the vicious red fog that clouds our minds.

Having to be honest with ourselves about *why* we really need anger is a very uncomfortable thing to do. We may find that it's because anger feels really good because it releases us from our conscience and our inhibitions.

For example, we may pride ourselves on being good people, and there is an internal cost to behaving in a way that doesn't reflect our own values, so there are certain things that we won't normally say or do. At work and in love, we are usually considerate in our words and actions because we value our relationships with others, both with work colleagues and partners in our personal lives. However, when we're *angry*, we suddenly find ourselves saying and doing things we wouldn't otherwise say or do; because when we're angry, the possible cost of our actions suddenly don't matter anymore.

Regardless of whether we're conscious of it or not, anger brings about a perceived sense of freedom, much like when we're drunk— we feel temporarily liberated. Drunken courage isn't real courage, and in the same way, anger isn't real power. When we're angry, we may lose our mind and only get it back much, much later, usually accompanied by regret. Because when we return to our rational mindset, we can clearly see the cost of our anger. That's not powerful—that is very sad.

Anger can gradually eat away at our quality of life while making us think it's enriching our existence. The more often we use anger as a tool, the more it dilutes the quality of our relationships and sets us further back as human beings.

When we look at why we get angry, it usually is because we feel like the situation is slipping away from us—when we can't understand something and don't agree with it, it feels like we have very little control over it. It's instinctive for us as human beings to turn to anger to try to wrestle back control.

Instilling fear is the easiest tool to use when we don't have other ways of making someone give us what we need. When we're fueled by anger, we usually feel justified to force compliance on someone. When people fear us, they don't question us. In that instant, it gives us an immense sense of power.

We think that we are using anger to empower ourselves, but the deeper truth is that we need anger to control people. Anger makes us feel better when we don't know how else to feel strong, to feel secure, to feel confident or good about ourselves. This is why the more insecure we are about ourselves, the more we feel we need to depend on the illusion of strength that anger brings.

Anger is not strength, because it is only when we are not capable or skilled that we will resort to using the *easiest* tool in our toolbox. When we need to use anger to instill fear as negative motivation to get others to do what we want, it's a sign that we don't know how else to resolve problems or how else to overcome our challenges in life.

This doesn't mean we are hopeless human beings—it just means that we have an opportunity to be honest and acknowledge that we need to *up our skills* in the areas of self-awareness and emotional resilience.

The purpose of acknowledging why and how we use anger isn't to make us to feel bad about ourselves, but for us to understand ourselves better. If we don't understand ourselves, we'll keep repeating the same behavior over the course of our lives without the realization that we are bringing more suffering into our lives and the lives of the people we love.

Is anger sometimes good? We'll have to ask ourselves if anger is giving us satisfaction or if it's bringing us happiness.

Is anger sometimes necessary? We'll think the answer is "yes" if we don't know any other way of solving problems. If there are no other tools in our toolbox, then anger will always be our only option, because it's the easiest. The reality is that there are many tools we can use to solve problems positively; and while anger can be used to motivate people to do what we want, it's certainly not a positive tool—not for our own state of mind and not for the people around us.

We need to develop other tools to use when standing up for ourselves or communicating with people we find difficult, because otherwise, we'll keep losing our minds over the smallest things. The more often we get angry, the more often we lose our mind to temporary insanity. This is self-inflicted suffering.

People may disagree with us or do things that hurt us, but only we can lose our own minds. If we're constantly unhappy with people, we have to look inwards to see if it's because we are still holding on to anger and the illusion of power it gives. We cannot let go of suffering if we cannot see how anger debilitates us and eats away at our quality of life.

PUT OUT THE FIRE;
DON'T ADD MORE FUEL TO IT

\<Understanding\>

Growing up, I witnessed my dad losing his temper over the smallest things. When he was in a state of fury, he would often shout so loudly that neighbors a few houses over could probably hear him.

When he was in that state of mind, my mom would stop talking. She wouldn't argue back or even point out how ridiculous he was being.

"Why don't you walk away? Or yell back?" I asked her a few times.

My mom raised me to stand up for myself, especially when I think I'm being bullied, and I couldn't understand why she wouldn't stand up for herself when my dad was clearly taking his anger out on her.

This was the time when I learned one of the most valuable lessons I ever learned from my mom—that there are many ways to stand up for ourselves, and we can do it in a way that *benefits* us the most. To do that, we have to be rational and strategic, which we cannot be if we *also* join in the madness of anger.

"If I shouted back at him or walked away, what would that achieve?" my mom asked me; "It would make him even more angry, and my objective is to *put out* the fire, not to add fuel to it."

My mom wasn't being passive, nor was she afraid of my dad. To her, it was simple—if someone is angry, her objective is to *not react* with anger. "If you're not adding fuel to the fire, you're not giving the person's anger anything to feed off of and it'll eventually sputter out. *Nobody can argue on their own.*"

What she said sounded so simple, but it really made me examine what my objectives were when I was having difficulty communicating with someone. Sometimes, we feel upset because *we're* trying to be nice and it's the *other person* who is arguing *with us!* Yet, logically, if we are not reacting with anger, how long can the other person argue on their own?

My mom's objective of putting out the fire when another person is angry *isn't* because she *agrees* with the person or what they're saying, but because she wants them to able to *hear* her when she speaks. "When someone is angry, whatever you want to say will go right over their heads. No one can hear a single word of what you say when they're angry, much less understand you."

That's so true—what is the point of wasting your effort in trying to talk to someone who is consumed by anger when they can't even hear, much less absorb, what you're saying?

This is why when someone is being irrational, my mom's objective is to put out the fire so that they can *return to rational thought*. Reacting with anger would only make things worse, which would bring her further away from her objective of not suffering.

So, where do we go from here? Does not reacting with anger mean that we're *supposed to be okay with everything?*

This was where I learned from my mom that anger is not the only tool to employ when standing up for ourselves and solving problems.

My dad wasn't physically violent when he lost his temper. If he had been, my mom would have immediately left the situation as well as exited the relationship both for her own and her children's safety. As it was, my mom was *never okay* with my dad's behavior—each time he lost his temper or behaved irrationally, my mom would pick a day and time to *bring up* the incident. Her goal was to make sure my father understood why his behavior was not acceptable so that he wouldn't do it again.

Contrary to how people usually "make" others behave, my mom was never accusatory in the way she spoke to my dad about his temper, nor was there blame or resentment. Her goal was to make sure my dad was in a state of mind where he was not defensive so that he had all the clarity in the world to think about his actions and why they weren't acceptable.

Because of how my mom communicated with him over the years, my father lost his temper less and less frequently until it hardly happened anymore. Since he couldn't get away with it, he had to learn how to communicate better instead of always just resorting to anger.

It's impossible to bully my mom—she won't let anyone get away with being unreasonable. Not only will she call you out on it, she has a way of explaining her logic to you that makes you feel incredibly aware of what you've done wrong. When it came to teaching my brother and I, she didn't need to punish us for us to feel remorseful—she just needed us to talk to us in a way that didn't make us feel defensive so we would reflect on our own behavior. I always joked that it would have been easier if she had punished us or yelled at us, because then we would have a reason to be angry at her instead of having to deal with our own consciences!

My mom has never believed in punishment, because she doesn't believe that fear will help us learn our lesson—fear doesn't actually teach people anything except how to never again get caught.

In life, of course we are not supposed to be "okay with everything." If someone is abusive or if we sense even an inkling of danger, we must take action to immediately exit the situation or relationship. Anger is *not an action,* which is why we cannot merely be angry at someone who is abusive toward us and feel that we have already taken action. Even if someone is sorry for being abusive, we still have to be able to find a way to exit the situation. This is why anger is so unnecessary, because it can *cloud our judgement* as to what is the best course of action to take to protect ourselves.

In life, if we find someone's behavior unacceptable, we must *always* take action to address it. Anger is never the best action to take, because actions taken in anger often bring us *further* away from our objectives.

There are so many instances in life where I feel like I want to be angry, but it's hard to stay angry when there's this voice in my head saying, "Xandria, you're making the situation worse."

Like my father, I used to use anger in my relationships, wielding it like the sharp tool that it is. I would shout when I felt like I couldn't find any other way to be heard, and I was a master in the art of the silent treatment. When I was angry, I would behave in the craziest and most irrational manner, and I would always be racked with guilt or shame afterwards.

But that still didn't stop me, because back then, I always felt so *justified* in "standing up for myself."

It wasn't until I took a good, hard look at myself in the mirror that I realized this wasn't the kind of person I wanted to be. This realization only came to me after my dad left, because I saw the grace and strength with which my mom handled the divorce. I admired that so much, and it finally hit me that there are much more effective ways to be strong and to stand up for ourselves than getting mired in anger.

Time and time again, my mom has shown me what *strength* means—it doesn't mean yelling back louder than someone else, or responding to anger with more anger. True strength is an emotional resilience that comes from knowing that we don't have to let circumstances and people dictate how we behave and respond. This way, we are able to take *better* action and solve problems more effectively.

When you think about it, we can be angry at someone for a very long time, yet the problem still doesn't get solved. Being angry not only doesn't fix the problem, it often turns it into a *bigger* problem.

WHEN WE'RE NOT DRIVEN BY OUR EGO, WE CAN LOSE THE BATTLE TO WIN THE WAR

<Self-Love>

Even when I realized that I didn't have to *participate in an argument* just to stand up for myself, I wasn't quite sure of *how* to do it—even when I truly didn't want to react negatively, I just didn't know *how* to not get angry.

It wasn't until I was willing to look inwards to understand myself better that I started figuring it out. To not react negatively, we have to understand where our reactions originate, and the source is often the ego. The ego is what causes us to seek external validation and significance, so it is where all our insecurities and doubts are amplified outwards. This is where we feel easily criticized, easily hurt, and easily angered because we take everything so personally.

Learning how to not get angry so easily is about learning how to accept ourselves so that we don't keep needing external validation to prove to ourselves how good or worthy we are as human beings. We don't react negatively when we don't take it personally, and that's only possible when we have a strong enough sense of self so that we are not attaching our sense of our own identity to other people's actions.

Self-acceptance and self-love can be seen as arrogance or as a way to excuse our own bad behavior, but in reality, it works exactly in the opposite manner. Accepting who we are is the very foundation of self-improvement, because it means we are not denying our flaws or trying to justify our weaknesses in an attempt to feel better about who we are.

If we love ourselves, we won't feel bad for being imperfect. We'll be able to *face* our flaws and weaknesses in a way that is kind and compassionate, rather than harsh and judgmental. It is when we are not judging our own fears and doubts that we have no need to blind ourselves to them. This is why acceptance and love for one's own self are so important, so we won't shy away from self-reflection.

When we don't really understand ourselves—our fears, needs, insecurities, and doubts—we will constantly be sensitive and reactive toward other people, which makes it hard not to be angry.

I've thought a lot about why my mom finds it easier than most people to refrain from reacting in anger, and I think it is because she has always had a very healthy self-esteem and a very small ego. She just naturally doesn't take things personally because she understands that people's anger is a manifestation of their pain and has nothing to do with her.

This is something that will be clear to all of us when we practice building a strong and healthy sense of self. With my mom, it's not that she doesn't feel anger, it's just that she can very quickly let go because she isn't driven by her ego to hold on to it. This frees her to think logically and find the best solution for her own objectives in every situation instead of letting people bait her into being unhappy.

More suffering comes when we are so driven by the ego—by our needs and fears—to win every little argument that we end up losing in the big picture. My mom often said to me, "Girl, sometimes, we have to lose the battle to win the war." And that's one of the wisest and most strategic pieces of advice to help us get what we want in life.

THERE ARE NO GOOD OR BAD EMOTIONS, ONLY THOSE THAT SERVE OR DON'T SERVE US

<Acceptance>

Understanding that holding on to anger and blame causes more suffering doesn't mean that we will immediately be able to let go of how we feel.

And if we cannot let go of what we want to release, it doesn't mean that we're "wrong." To be human is to experience a range of emotions. There is no right and wrong when it comes to how we feel—we feel what we feel, and that's the reality of it.

It is in the nature of human beings to want to put things into boxes—this is good, this is bad; this is right, and this is wrong. Perhaps a more useful alternative would be to examine what is helpful and what is not helpful.

If what we feel brings us more peace, it's helpful, because it serves our objective of being happy.

If what we feel brings us more suffering, it's unhelpful, because it doesn't serve our objective of being happy.

In light of this, distinctions like good versus bad and right versus wrong don't matter as much as what is helpful or unhelpful to our objectives in life. Negative emotions are not bad emotions—we only identify some emotions as negative because it is a signal to ourselves of what we want to be able to release.

The reason why it's so important not to label or judge our emotions is because instead of letting go of our negative emotions, we'll be trying to get *rid* of them. It's deeply instinctive for us to try to get rid of something that we think is "bad."

"Letting go" of an emotion is not the same as "getting rid of" it. The former brings acceptance and compassion, whereas the latter brings resentment and harshness. Trying to *rid ourselves* of anything suggests that we have ill will toward it, and that we have ill will toward ourselves. It means that we are judging ourselves for the negativity we feel, so now besides the original feeling of unhappiness, there's also this secondary unhappiness that's gaining momentum.

For this reason, when we try to get rid of our negative emotions, it usually results in us feeling even more frustrated because we feel like we're trying so hard, yet we don't feel better.

Any negative emotion, such as anger or sadness, is like a train. When a train is moving, you can't just slam your foot down on the brake to stop it. We cannot force a thing to stop happening by trying to bend it to our will.

This is why it's important to understand that letting go of our negative emotions is not about controlling how we feel—letting go is the *opposite* of control. It's very hard to control water sloshing about in a glass by holding the glass more and more tightly. For water to be still, we just have to put the glass down and *let it be.*

It is only when we are not fighting against something that it stops being difficult for us. It is only when we can accept who we are that we can move past what we don't like about ourselves.

Accepting our negative emotions is not the same as giving ourselves permission to continue on a path of self-pity; it isn't about excusing ourselves, nor does it mean that it's justifiable to project our negative emotions onto the people around us.

Accepting our negative emotions doesn't mean behaving negatively, it means we stop compounding the difficulty in stressful situations. When we engage in this kind of acceptance, we acknowledge the emotions that are not helpful to our lives and we move ourselves toward the step of letting them go. It does not mean we are pretending to be happy or that our negative emotions aren't there.

Life is either a celebration or a lesson, so when we feel negative emotions, we can use them as a *signal* as to what it wants us to *learn* about ourselves. To do that, we have to acknowledge how we feel, and most importantly, allow ourselves to feel the emotion in all its uncomfortable glory.

When you don't like what you're feeling, what *message* is your emotion trying to tell you about your self-esteem and your ego? What action does it want you to take that brings more happiness and less suffering to your life? How does it want to you learn and evolve as a person?

As mentioned in chapter one, there is no need for self-criticism in our journey of self-improvement. It's not necessary to beat ourselves up for our own imperfections and weaknesses—because that is not the lesson.

The lesson is self-compassion.

We need to learn and grow, and all our negative emotions are there to help us learn how to evolve into being kinder people—and to learn to be kind to ourselves even when it's hard. If we can do that, we can also be kind to others even when it's hard.

When we can be compassionate toward ourselves, we can be compassionate toward others. It is only when we practice a nonjudgmental approach to ourselves that we will truly understand what it means to refrain from judging others for how they feel.

We don't have to define our emotions and label them as "good" or "bad." Instead, we can practice letting go of what is not helpful and not useful to our happiness. We can let go of what doesn't serve us.

DON'T USE BLAME AND GUILT
TO PUNISH YOURSELF

<Acceptance>

It's common and perhaps natural for us to blame ourselves when we've made a horrible mistake or done something we regret. Blaming ourselves is almost like a punishment we think we deserve because we feel so bad about what happened. Blame is often accompanied by feelings of guilt, which we may even *welcome*, because we may feel we *should* live with the burden after doing something that we regret.

We often feel that blaming ourselves is a sign that we're taking responsibility, but what blame actually does is sit inside us and may even immobilize us. The danger of blame and guilt is that we'll feel we've taken action in response to our mistakes when in actual fact, we've done nothing except feel bad. Feeling bad doesn't make us better people.

Responsibility, on the other hand, is active—it empowers us to admit our mistakes and shines a light for us to see how we can do better. Blame and guilt keep taking us back into the past because we keep reliving our mistakes over and over again, but responsibility brings us into the future—it gives us hope and an action plan for how we can change things.

Without blame, there is only "what has happened." It is neither good nor bad. There is no need to judge the situation, and more importantly, no need to judge yourself. With this awareness, there is no regret. When we are not consumed by regrets, we are able to think more honestly and take responsibility for the consequences that come with our actions.

Punishing ourselves causes more suffering. We may believe we deserve to suffer because we want to atone our mistakes, but how is our suffering helping us put right what we have done wrong?

Again, taking responsibility and doing something about it in the world are active, and blame and guilt are passive.

If we really want to pay a penance, we can choose to do the more challenging thing, and what is harder than voluntarily suffering is to learn how to take responsibility for our own happiness. This means not only acknowledging our weaknesses, but *taking action* toward growth in self-awareness and emotional maturity, which is significantly *harder* than choosing to live with blame and guilt.

This is why when it comes to mistakes, we have to learn how to take responsibility without beating ourselves up. If we are distracted or blinded by the need to punish ourselves, we won't have the clarity to identify our weaknesses and be honest with ourselves about how we can be better.

We cannot go backward, only forward. When you've done something you wish you could take back, the best thing to do is not to carry a heavy burden of guilt around. What is done cannot be undone, what is said cannot be unsaid. Where there is hurt, it can never be taken back. Where there has been betrayal, it can never be undone; but what is in the *future* is yet to be determined. One can always take full responsibility for the mistakes we regret having made by being even more determined to grow positively as a person. We may not be able to erase the hurt we have caused, but we can make it our purpose to bring joy to the lives of the people we meet in the future, and this requires knowing how to be a happy person.

If we are harsh and unforgiving toward ourselves, we will also be harsh and unforgiving toward others. If we cannot accept ourselves, we cannot accept others—and that's double suffering. If we cannot let go of our own suffering, we will always absorb more suffering.

When we adopt a non-blame mindset toward ourselves, it becomes easier to adopt a non-blame mindset toward other people, and by doing so, we are consciously choosing not to be weighed down and essentially removing a huge part of what blocks our happiness.

HATE SPILLS OVER TO THE PEOPLE WE LOVE, ESPECIALLY OUR CHILDREN

<Awareness>

The anger and blame that we carry with us in our everyday lives doesn't just affect our own mental health and happiness, it also affects the lives of the people closest to us—our family members and those we love.

When we cannot let go of anger and hatred, our children will absorb our bitterness and suffering into their own lives. And they will carry this burden through their own adult life, and it will impact the way they solve problems in their own relationships.

When parents speak ill of each other to their children, the children won't know what to do with the information. Out of loyalty to one parent, they will often adopt the same anger and judgement toward the other parent.

Kids who are constantly exposed to their parents complaining about one another or arguing with each other will likely grow up normalizing anger—they'll think that when you love someone, it's "healthy" to also hate them a little.

This is why it's even *more* important for us to learn how to let go when we have children.

If one's relationship with one's partner doesn't work out, it doesn't matter whose fault it is, because what matters more is that we understand the importance of not holding on to anger or hate.

When you feel hurt and wronged, it's human nature to want your family to take your side and support you, but we often don't realize how deep of an imprint our insecurities and fears will leave on our children—it'll manifest in their relationships when they have their own family. This is one of the key reasons why so many kids grow into adults who find it difficult to be happy in their relationships yet don't know why.

How parents bring up their children is a result of how they feel about themselves and their lives. If parents don't know how to take responsibility for their own happiness, if they often blame one another for their misery, or if they often use anger and fear as tools for getting what they want, then there is a very high chance that their approach to life will impact their children's approach to life.

When my father left my mother and married the woman with whom he was having an affair, my brother and I could draw our own conclusions about our father's behavior and actions without our perceptions being colored by the need to take sides or to "protect" our mom.

We both chose not to keep in touch with our dad for our own reasons, not because we felt pressured to take sides or because we blamed him for what happened. We don't agree with his actions, but we understand that it wasn't because we weren't worthy of love that he did what he did. We didn't feel rejected or unloved— our decision was based on our own beliefs and what we could or could not respect.

However, if my mom had harbored anger or resentment toward my dad, my brother and I would likely have taken on what she was feeling; and whether we were conscious of it or not, anger and resentment toward our father *would* have impacted our lives, because negative emotions we carry manifest into neediness and fear in our *own* relationships.

If our mother had suffered, we would also have suffered. But because our mother never viewed herself as a victim, my brother and I never viewed ourselves that way, either.

This is one of the biggest reasons why we need to let go of anger and blame—it stops us from thinking and feeling like victims. If we go through life believing that we are victims, then life will always treat us like we are. If we have suffered at the hands of someone and we are not willing let go of anger and blame, then we have to be aware of the negative consequences that may arise—bitterness weighs us *and* our families down. When we're not happy, it's likely that nobody around us will find it easy to be happy.

We let go and forgive people for our own happiness, but we *also* do it for the quality of life of the people we love.

Don't let your legacy to your family be one of anger and hate.

WHAT IS IT FROM OUR PAST THAT WEIGHS US DOWN TODAY?

<Self-Love>

If you think that something in your childhood or your upbringing is holding you back from being able to feel good about yourself and your life, there is only one thing to do—let go of it.

Let go of the blame, anger, and guilt of the past. The way we are brought up has a huge impact on us and can condition how we think and feel about ourselves. And as long as we cannot let go of the negativity or hurt from the past, it will constantly be a weight we carry with us no matter how hard we try to build a good life for ourselves today. We have to free ourselves from the pain of the past so that we live our lives with the happiness we want.

This is easier said than done, but if there is anything worth spending our time and effort on doing, it is this. The circumstances that shaped our lives growing up may not have been up to us—we cannot choose our parents or our caretakers, and we certainly have no power over their decisions as to how they bring us up—but we can definitely make our own decisions at the present moment of how we want our lives to be.

Our trauma and suffering may not be our fault, but our happiness is always our own responsibility. This doesn't mean that we discount the hurt and pain caused by the people who should know how to love us, it means that we take back the power of our own quality of life.

Life can present us with many challenges, but many of the struggles we face are internal struggles. The primary barriers to our happiness aren't the jobs we didn't get or the relationships that didn't work out; the real barrier is how we *feel* about ourselves in the midst of it all.

Why is it that, as adults who have successful careers and loving families of our own, we can still have a chip on our shoulders or such a void in our lives? Why is it that no matter how old we get, we still have such a need for acceptance, validation, and significance?

When we examine why we expect so much from ourselves and our lives and why we find it so hard to accept ourselves and to be happy, we may find that much of what holds us back is an outgrowth of the experiences we've had growing up.

When we examine our needs and fears, we can see that there is a deep instinctual need inside almost every one of us for love and acceptance. It is human nature to want to be seen, accepted, and loved by the people we admire. Most of the time, we want love, respect, and acceptance from our parents, but it could be anyone from our childhood years—an aunt or uncle, a sibling, or any parental figure in our lives who was part of our upbringing.

Our relationships with the people from whom we want and need love and acceptance drive the way we think and feel about ourselves—more often than not, what our parents believe about us forms our own beliefs of who we are as adults. How we see ourselves then drives our ability or inability to feel fulfilled in our lives.

For example, if our parents compared us to other kids when we were growing up, we are likely to have subconsciously picked up the message that in order to be deserving of love and approval, we need to be better than others. As an adult, this can manifest either in our being insecure about ourselves because we think we're not good enough, or in our being arrogant because we constantly think that we need to be better than others to be deserving.

Arrogance can be a self-inflated perception of who we are, but when you think about it, arrogance comes from a *need* to be better than others; this need comes from the belief that if we're not better than they are, it means that we are not worthy. People don't *set out* to be arrogant, just like people don't set out to be insecure—they are both the *result* of our need to prove to ourselves that we are deserving, significant, and worthy. Arrogance and insecurity are two sides of the same coin, because they both come from the same source, a need for external significance and validation This is a set of perceptions that we most likely learned through the experiences we had with our parents in our growing years.

Some parents use anger and criticism as a tool to motivate their children to do better. This sends a message that anger and criticism is love. Some parents use punishment as a tool to motivate their children to be good. This normalizes the concept of guilt and blame.

Some parents are careful not to praise their kids in order to keep them humble, so as adults, they never feel quite deserving no matter what they achieve.

At the other extreme, some parents think their children can do no wrong, so as adults, they tend to go through life viewing themselves as victims because they think the problems in their lives are caused by other people.

Some parents have a few kids, and it can be harder to ensure that every single child *feels* loved in the way they need; so children with many siblings may grow up doubting themselves or trying harder to prove themselves because deep down, they may believe that they are less worthy of love and attention. This has been called "middle child syndrome," although in reality, *all kinds* of syndromes exist based on the different experiences we have growing up.

Concepts like 'rejection' have no meaning in our vocabulary until we actually experience what they feel like. As children, we learn very quickly to adapt to the people around us with a single objective—to be loved and praised, and to please others and prevent ourselves from being rejected. But if we cannot have love or praise, we will settle for attention.

We often don't know at what point in our lives we subconsciously picked up cues on what to do and how to conduct ourselves to get more love and to avoid rejection. This manifests in our behaving in all sorts of ways to get approval and to feel significant, and as adults, we *still operate* in a very similar way, just toward different things.

These threads from our past shape so much of our present, yet they can rarely be seen on the surface and often only emerge when we have our own relationships and careers, especially when we struggle to find fulfilment.

Where do our self-limiting beliefs come from?

Why do we feel intimidated or inferior in the presence of people who are successful?

Why are we defensive or reactive toward people who challenge us?

Why do we criticize ourselves and then become so harsh toward others?

Why do we hold on so tightly to righteousness and power?

Why do we link our happiness to what we have or don't have?

Why do we link our self-worth to who loves or doesn't love us?

Why is it so hard to be fulfilled, even when we know we have a lot going for us?

As human beings, we may seem extremely complicated on the surface, but when we look deeper, all our internal struggles are driven by very simple and similar needs and fears—the need to be accepted, to be loved, and to be significant…and the fear that we are not.

Our sense of self-worth as adults is tightly tied to the people from whom we most crave love and respect. If they have said or done anything that leaves us feeling rejected in the form of criticism, comparison, neglect, or betrayal, it can be very hard for us to *believe* in our own worth as human beings.

This is why self-acceptance and self-love are so difficult, because if the very people who are supposed to love us cannot love us, then deep down in our psyches, it's very easy to believe that there must be something wrong with us.

Even if you have chosen not to keep in touch with your parents, even if you can see how flawed or toxic the people you love are, you may still go through life seeking the validation and acceptance you felt you never had, because deep down inside, you might still believe that there's something wrong with you that caused the people you love to reject you.

If we feel that our parents have disappointed us or let us down in our past, it's really important for our happiness in the *present* day to let go of any anger or resentment that we carry with us about that.

If we feel that our parents have not been able to accept us, it's important to let go of the belief that our worth is tied to their acceptance of us.

In order to be free from the pain of the past, we have to first accept and forgive the people who have intentionally or unintentionally hurt us in our childhood. The scars or traumas we accumulated when we were growing up are definitely not our fault, but we have to be able to choose to let go of what doesn't serve us.

Choosing to let go of pain or trauma from the past can be an extremely difficult practice in itself, which is why it is easier to escape physically and never look back. It is not necessary to look back to the point that we relive the past, but it is necessary to be able to look inwards to acknowledge our hurt and pain, to *forgive* the people who have hurt us, and then to let it go.

This was the very difficult process a friend of mine had to go through when she forgave her brother for sexually abusing her when they were children. My friend is a positive person, and it wasn't that she was unhappy with life, but she told me that she had never felt *truly free* to live with absolute joy. For years during her adult life, the trauma impacted her relationships, and it was always something heavy inside of her. So years later, she at last chose to do something about it—to acknowledge the full extent of the pain and betrayal she felt and go through the painful process of having an honest conversation with her brother about it. It was one of the most difficult things she had ever done, but she did not avoid it. She realized that as an adult, she could *choose* the story of her life—she was no longer helpless or hopeless. She genuinely forgave her brother, and I can only imagine how hard it must have been for her to go through the process needed to arrive at a place of genuine forgiveness. Undertaking this was an acknowledgement to herself that she wasn't unworthy or incapable—that what happened wasn't her fault, and that although her brother's actions had caused her pain, she chose not to blame him, because that would have been suffering she would have had to carry with her. It wasn't in any way easy for her to forgive and let go, but it was the kind of challenge that was completely worth facing.

It is only when we are completely absent of even the tiniest bit of resentment or blame toward those we believe are supposed to love us that we will be completely free to be happy. This is the only way to be free of any self-limiting beliefs, because as long as we cannot let go, we will be holding on to voices from the past telling us that we will never be enough.

If the people we love say or do things that imply we are worthless, it is up to us to *see our own worth*. If people we love cannot love and accept us, it is up to us to work twice as hard to *love and accept ourselves*, which means we have to work doubly hard to acknowledge and let go of what doesn't serve us.

When we truly believe in our own worth, we are able to stop projecting our needs and fears onto the people around us. Then we won't be afraid to stand up for ourselves for fear of rejection, nor will we constantly seek to please people because of our need for love and acceptance.

To be happy, we need to be able to recognize the patterns of our suffering and discern whether there are any burdens we are carrying from our childhood that are holding us back. It is only when we work on letting go of the pain of the past that we won't seek happiness externally in an unconscious way to try to fill a void in our lives, be it in our careers or in love.

WE CANNOT LET GO
OF WHAT WE PRETEND
ISN'T THERE

<Acceptance>

Letting go is probably one of the hardest practices in the world, because letting go is an internal practice that requires us to see and understand ourselves. It's really hard to understand why we can be so deeply affected by people and circumstances; and it's challenging to be honest about our needs and fears. It's also hard to value and love ourselves in such a way that the ego no longer needs to seek external comfort, assurance, or validation.

Letting go is daunting; it can feel nearly impossible, especially when we've been hurt or when we're angry. Letting go can feel torturous, and when we look at it, when it feels that painful, it's usually because we are trying to suppress how we feel. Suppressing how we feel is something that many of us have instinctively managed to grasp, because we learn early on in life that we can't just throw tantrums or lose our tempers in public, at work, or even at home. But this suppression also causes all our frustration and anger to accumulate and build up somewhere inside of us, where one day, like an overfull dam, it overflows and we have to let it all out. This usually doesn't bode so well for us, either for our own stress levels or for our relationships with other people.

This is where it really helps to understand that letting go isn't about controlling or suppressing how we feel. Letting go is never about invalidating our emotions or pretending that they're not there. It's the opposite—letting go is about being fully present with how we are feeling, because it is only when we can *look* at our pain that it can slowly recede. We cannot let go of something that is so deeply buried or that we are pretending isn't there.

Also, it's not like letting go is something we do once and then we're over it all and never feel affected ever again. Someone once said to me, "The work is within ourselves. Letting go is the process of keeping the heart clean and keeping the heart open."

When you think about it, keeping the heart clean is pretty much like keeping a house clean—it's *constant work*. We don't clean the house just once, feel proud of ourselves, and then expect it to stay perfect all the time; nor do we get frustrated when dirt comes in.

When the house isn't as clean as we would like it to be, we just get to cleaning again.

Sometimes, we need to practice letting go of the *same* thing over and over again.

We're human, and being human means that it's hard to truly understand ourselves—sometimes we think we've let go, but then later discover that it still bothers us, which is an indication that perhaps we haven't fully let go. Instead of feeling frustrated or denying the truth of how we feel, we can go through the practice of letting go again.

What does this practice mean, exactly?

The practice of letting go is the practice of understanding ourselves so that we are able to recognize when we're feeling negatively charged—and then, instead of quickly suppressing that uncomfortable feeling, burying it somewhere down deep, or pretending we're not affected by it, we acknowledge what we're feeling.

So much of the practice of letting go requires one very simple thing: the ability to sit in discomfort. Our self-protection mechanisms almost always kick in to shield us from what is uncomfortable—this is why denial is such a common coping mechanism—and our instinctive reaction is to immediately try to alleviate any discomfort or pain we feel. This is the primary reason why denial, suppressing our feelings, or blocking out what bothers us are almost always our first reactions. We do these things so automatically that we may not even be aware of them.

For me, it was a slow process of becoming aware of how valuable the state of being uncomfortable can be. I've always wanted to be a better person, but I didn't realize that my knee-jerk reaction to any discomfort was to immediately alleviate the pain—either by lashing out in anger or distracting myself with happier things.

It took me a long time to realize that the only way to actually *become* a better person is to *grow,* and that the best way to grow is to be in a state of discomfort—how can we grow if we're always comfortable? This is why the path of least resistance is hardly ever the most rewarding—not having any resistance in life doesn't automatically bring fulfilment. *Growth* brings fulfilment. Ironically, for us as human beings, it is not when things are perfect that we are the most happy—it is when we are filled with purpose that we are the most happy. And when we ask ourselves what gives us purpose in life, the answer is usually linked to self-discovery and growth. Human beings fear death, but we probably fear stagnation even more.

To sit with discomfort, first we need to be able to look at our own pain without suppression or denial. This is where we begin to understand ourselves better, and this is where we find true comfort and solace—we can only *distract* ourselves from discomfort and pain when we seek soothing comfort and solace from external sources like people and things.

I've always wanted to be a more patient person. But it wasn't until I realized the value of sitting with discomfort that I understood that we cannot *try to be more patient*, because patience is not something we can force ourselves to feel—patience is what we learn when we are willing to sit in discomfort instead of reacting to alleviate the discomfort.

I truly believe that the practice of letting go will help us discover more about ourselves, which will bring us to a place where we simply are not disturbed or affected by anything or anyone. This sounds incredible, even impossible, because we're human, after all. But people who are never affected by outside stressors aren't weird or strange, rather it is that they are able to live with the deepest empathy, understanding, and acceptance because they can see the *truth* of things—that no one is our enemy, least of all ourselves.

Many of us can understand this, but not all of us can *live* it yet. This is why there is a practice for everything, but especially for letting go.

TO LET GO OF THE BIG THINGS, PRACTICE LETTING GO OF THE SMALL, EVERYDAY THINGS

<Understanding>

My mom, who can let go more quickly and easily than anyone I know, says, "It's not that I don't feel affected, it's about how quickly can I let go when I feel affected."

My best friend Sue, who can react just like anyone else, has an incredible capacity to be truly happy, says almost the same thing: "I get mad for like ten seconds, and then I get over it." I remember both of us laughing when she said that, but it basically summed up the practice of letting go.

It is likely that we will feel a negative charge each time something bothers us. The question is, what are we going to do about it? Hold on because we feel righteous? Suppress it because we want to control how we feel? Bury it somewhere down deep so we don't have to deal with feeling uncomfortable? Or acknowledge how we feel so that we can decide what the best course of action is?

When I feel upset or weighed down, the tool that I use to determine what steps to take next is to ask myself, "Do I want to suffer?"—and sometimes, when I'm feeling particularly angry and in pain, my inner voice will yell, "Yes!"

It's interesting how when we are agitated, the ego takes over and tells us we *need* to be in pain to make the hurt we are feeling *matter*—we are tricked into thinking we are not suffering when we clearly are. However, the moment we become aware of this, our true sense of self can emerge, which means our rational mind is once again the main driver behind our decisions. This is when we can ask ourselves, "Do I want to suffer?" and the answer will be a quiet "No."

For someone who has a lot of practice, like my mom, the answer is always "No." All she has to do is focus on her objective and she can truly let something go.

Non-suffering is not the same as pleasure—in fact, as previously mentioned, we have to first allow ourselves to sit with discomfort to truly understand and acknowledge what we are feeling so that we can let go. Otherwise, we'll distract ourselves from the discomfort or alleviate our pain externally, so that what is affecting us just gets absorbed into us and becomes another burden we are unwittingly carrying around.

Because of this, even the little irritations, annoyances, and frustrations we experience are like little chunks of baggage—small parcels that come in with the delivery man that slowly accumulate into one giant burden.

Is it any wonder that we may feel unfulfilled and unhappy with life?

What can help us let go of the heavy burdens and difficult challenges in our lives is to practice letting go of the small things on a day-to-day basis—so we can learn how to recognize the small things that affect us and choose not to toss them onto the load we're carrying, but instead, let them go.

On any day when we feel a negative charge inside ourselves, we can practice recognizing it, acknowledging it, and then making a decision to change the trajectory of our feelings. To begin this practice, examine what your "normal" reactions are to something that bothers you and decide to respond differently the next time it happens. For example, if you notice that you are always upset by rude drivers, make it a conscious decision to *respond differently* the next time it happens—if you always swear, change it to a smile. If you always honk loudly, change it to turning on the radio. It's not about suppressing how you feel, but rather recognizing what you do out of habit and asking yourself if you want to continue *taking on* these small miseries and adding them to what already weighs you down.

Can reading a disagreeable email make us upset? Does being in
a traffic jam put us in a bad mood? Will a difficult talk with our
partner ruin our weekend? Do we automatically have a bad day
when something undesirable happens? When we're unhappy, do
we carry the vibe of negativity with us through our day and pass it
on to the people we meet?

This is what letting go is—a constant practice of checking in with
ourselves to examine what baggage we might be carrying so that
we can put it down.

Nobody *wants* to be in a bad mood. It's not our intention to be
easily annoyed and quick to anger, and most of the time we're
not conscious of the impact that all this accumulated suffering
will have on us. This is because on the surface, we don't see our
grumpiness, impatience, and bad moods as pain or suffering. It's
not that big a deal because we're not *un*happy.

However, not being unhappy is not happiness, either. This is why
we can have so much going for us yet feel lost or unfulfilled. One
may be grateful, and one may have a good job and a wonderful
family, so why then would one ever feel unfulfilled? It's like we can
be happy on a day-to-day basis, yet at the same time, we may feel
like we don't *have* happiness.

One of the main reasons why we may feel this way is because the
small accumulated burdens that we cannot release solidify into
very solid barriers to our happiness.

If we are not in the practice of letting go of the small things, it's
very hard to let go of the big things. If we don't work out on a
regular basis, we won't have the capacity to be able to be strong
when the occasion calls for it. This is why letting go of the small,
everyday things that bother us is such an important practice,
because with each small challenge comes the opportunity to
practice lifting some weights. Letting go of the hurt that people
have caused us or the pain we've experienced in our life is not
easy because the *weight* of it is so heavy, but we can do it—if we
put in the work to build our muscles.

Yuri and I like to joke that happiness is like working out, but instead of working on our abs, we're building our six-pack of happiness! Life doesn't get easier, *we get stronger.*

The more we practice non-suffering on a day-to-day basis, the easier letting go becomes for us, especially when the big challenges come our way.

CHAPTER FIVE

Living with Joy, Positivity, and Gratitude

FOR WHEN YOU WANT TO GROW:

PRACTICE THE THREE STAGES OF HAPPINESS—THE REHEARSAL, THE PERFORMANCE, AND THE REVIEW

<Understanding>

Even when something makes complete sense to us, it doesn't mean that it's easy.

It can be extremely frustrating when we feel like we're not making much progress despite *wanting* to do better. It is even more frustrating when we've put in a great deal of effort yet still find ourselves unable to improve our relationships, let go of stress at work, or stop worrying about what people think of us.

We may put a ton of effort into self-improvement—reading books, attending workshops, and genuinely wanting to accept, let go, and remove the barriers to our happiness—yet it can still be hard to be happy.

One of the main reasons why we feel frustrated when life is hard is because we forget that happiness is not the default human state. Whether consciously or subconsciously, we see happiness as our default emotion, as if "happy" is how we *should be*. So when we're not happy, we feel frustrated because we feel we're not living life as we "should be" living it.

Part of the reason why happiness feels like the default state is because happiness used to come so easily to us—most of us have memories, however deeply submerged, of the blissful state of contentment that we experienced as infants.

However, as babies, we are all easily happy, not because we have no challenges, but because the challenges in a baby's life are pretty much limited to hunger and staying warm, and *somebody* is always there to solve those problems for us. Every time we're hungry, we're fed and the problem is resolved.

As we grow older, many other factors start coming into play—we have challenges at work, challenges in our relationships, challenges with family, and even challenges within our own mind. So, as adults, not only are our challenges much more daunting, there's also no one to help solve them for us—nobody is there to remove the barriers to our happiness, so we have to learn how to do it ourselves.

However, because happiness was neither something we had to consciously learn growing up nor a subject taught in school, it might not occur to us as adults that we have to acquire various tools for happiness and *practice* them in order to maintain or heighten our level of happiness. This is why life feels so difficult when we're unhappy—we think that happiness shouldn't be that hard or that life is not fair. However, that's not the case— happiness is just a practice, and any kind of practice is hard.

It is when the practice of happiness is extremely frustrating that we have to remind ourselves of one thing: It's precisely because it is a *practice* that almost everything is easier said than done. Don't give up or be hard on yourself on the days when you're not able to be the best version of yourself.

When it comes to sports or art, we understand that we have to practice in order to get better. When the practice is hard and frustrating, we don't think, *Bah! It's easier said than done!* and give up—we work even harder to improve our skills.

When learning to ski or play the piano, it's very easy to understand and accept that our *intention* is not the same as our *ability*. Just because we want to take up the activity doesn't mean we'll have the skills to do it, much less excel at it when we begin. However, when it comes to our practice in the pursuit of happiness—for which we have to do lots of emotional heavy lifting, such as understanding our own emotions and triggers, learning not to react negatively, and letting go—we have a tendency to subconsciously feel that having good intentions *is* ability.

For this reason, it can be really frustrating when we are trying hard to be happy—since we know we have the intention, *why* aren't we progressing? It's because intention is *not* ability. Just because we come to realize something doesn't mean we have the ability to immediately create change.

If you've noticed, movies tend to perpetuate the belief that, when we have good intentions, we're *already* a better person. For example, when the hero in a movie *realizes* something, it is like a switch is flipped and he or she is suddenly this kind, generous, amazing, and loving person!

But that's not how it happens in real life—awareness is wonderful, but it doesn't mean we suddenly have ability. When we're aware, it helps us take a step in the *right direction* toward where we want to go. After awareness, there are many steps to take—we have to *close the gap* between intention and ability, and that takes practice which isn't going to be easy.

Because of all this, growing as a person takes conscious practice. The saying "Another year older, another year wiser" isn't necessarily true—the passing of time doesn't necessarily make us wiser or happier unless we make a conscious effort to grow.

Ever since I was a teenager, I've wanted to make sure my mom feels loved. However, that was easier said than done—I definitely love her, but does she *feel* loved or special? Even though I tried not to be impatient around my mom, I almost always ended up being impatient anyway, especially when I was tired or busy. The tone of my voice or my reactions would come across as inconsiderate or flippant. I constantly felt frustrated and guilty—why couldn't I treat the most precious person in my life with the esteem and love that matched what I felt for her?

One day, my husband saw how bad I was feeling after being out with my mom; despite my good intentions, I had ended up being impatient with her yet again.

"It's okay," he assured me, "At least you're aware."

And then it hit me. This wasn't *awareness*, this was *hindsight*. I was always having hindsights when it came to my mom—I would always *realize later* what I could have done better. Having realizations is better than *not* having any realizations, but realizations without change always just ends up being hindsight. And all these insights—too little and too late—were going to add up to huge regrets in the future.

This was when it hit me again—for so many years, I had been putting so much effort into trying to be patient with my mom. But if I am not a patient *person*, how could I be miraculously patient when I was in her presence? I would just be trying to control my impatience, which was why it was always a struggle.

It's the same thing with *everything* else—if one is not a calm and understanding person, it's impossible to be calm and understanding even when one wants to communicate positivity. This is how even when we try *so hard* not to be angry or lose our tempers, we can't help but react negatively when a difficult situation arises.

When everything is going well and we are in the best of moods, then there's no problem with being the best version of ourselves. But when we're busy, stressed, tired, or annoyed, we're always going to revert to our *habitual behavior*.

Often, when we encounter difficult situations, we're on autopilot. For example, if we work in customer service, it's easy to smile and be cheerful when everything is going well. But when it's really busy and we're stressed, we'll be operating on autopilot mode—we don't have time to think or plan, we'll just do what is habitual for us to do.

This goes for every single scenario, whether it's with our kids and family members at home, with our colleagues and clients at work, or with strangers whom we happen to come across over the course of a day. If we're impatient people, it's hard to be calm when we're stressed. If we're sensitive and defensive, it's hard to listen or communicate when we're upset. If we're prone to anger, it's hard not to say or do things we'll later regret.

Often, our autopilot responses create a great deal of unhappiness for ourselves and for the people we love. When we consciously practice happiness, it means we are working on *changing our habitual responses* so that when we default to our autopilot mode, we're operating from a calm and kind state of mind.

For more than ten years, I had good intentions of being a better person, but I was still making little to no progress when it came to being patient and loving toward my mom when I was tired or stressed. That was when I decided that I couldn't just depend on my mood or my luck or my control—I had to genuinely grow as a person and transform the aspects of myself that didn't serve me. It is not the intention but the *practice of happiness* that creates change.

For me, the practice of happiness can be divided into three stages.

STAGE ONE: THE REHEARSAL

This stage is where I work on understanding myself—everything that was mentioned in the first four chapters helps tremendously during this stage.

Stage one is about acceptance instead of control, understanding ourselves instead of suppressing who we are, being willing to be honest in identifying and acknowledging what we have to work on, and, most importantly, it's about *applying* it across all areas of our lives.

Just like a performance, the majority of the work is done *before* the show, because, when the show starts, you don't have time to think—your movements will be based on what you've rehearsed. How well we respond to a challenging situation depends on the work we've put in *beforehand*—if we haven't put in the work to develop an understanding of ourselves and other people, we will not be aware of our triggers and sensitivities, and that means it will be very hard for us *not* to react negatively in a difficult situation.

And here's the thing—during every stage show, unexpected glitches and problems will occur. This is one of the main reasons why it's so important to be well-rehearsed, because if there's a wrench thrown into the works, there won't be much time to think. We'll have to react instinctively, and we want to be so practiced that our instinctive response is one that will help us and not make things worse.

The same principle applies to life as a whole; when something unexpected happens, we react. This is why it's called a *reaction*— we automatically respond in the way that is habitual for us. For example, even when we tell ourselves we want to communicate positivity in our relationship, the moment our partner says something that feels unexpectedly hurtful, it hits us like a ton of bricks. It is precisely at this moment that we need to draw on the tools that we've been practicing in our everyday lives—including pretty much everything in Chapters 2 and 3, especially the mindset of not taking things personally—so that we can convey to our partner how much it hurts instead of accusing them of hurting us.

So don't practice happiness *only* during on certain occasions or only around the people who are important to you—because that's not enough practice. We need to practice recognizing our own ego, our sensitivities, and our triggers on a day-to-day basis with *everyone*, including the waiter at lunch, the mail carrier who comes to the door, the colleague who rubs us the wrong way, and even the driver who cuts us off on the road.

Don't "turn it on" only when you have an important meeting with clients or with the people you love, because that won't improve how you tend to respond to situations. We're not progressing when we only master controlling ourselves and our emotions because when something unexpected happens, we'll always lose control and revert right back to our habitual responses.

For this reason, it's also important to practice when things are going well, when we're in a good mood, and when what we face are just small annoyances and irritations—because, just like a good rehearsal, it'll prepare us for the challenges that lie ahead.

STAGE TWO: THE PERFORMANCE

This is showtime. When we're in a *very challenging* situation, we get to *apply* the strength we've gained from the work we've done in stage one.

All the muscles we've built by letting go of the little miseries can really help us now that it's time to lift the heavy weights. When we're upset, we'll know how to focus on our objectives and not get carried away with righteous anger, because we've done it on a daily basis. When we're down or depressed, we'll know how to not judge or blame ourselves, because, by then, we will understand that judgement and blame are not necessary to grow as a person. When we're triggered, we'll know how to not take it personally and how to communicate positively, because we'll have done it before.

When we've done something repeatedly, we can raise the level of our habitual responses a notch or two so that when we're operating on autopilot during stressful situations, we'll be better at communicating or problem-solving than before.

This is why every single difficult situation is an *opportunity* for us—because again, if we don't have these moments that really challenge us, how can we measure how far we've come? When you and your partner argue or experience conflict, don't view it as something unpleasant, but instead see it as a positive opportunity to understand yourself and understand your partner better.

When you are in a bad mood, see it as an opportunity to lift yourself up by putting your new practices of positivity into motion. When you are hurt or in pain, see it as an opportunity to practice acceptance and letting go.

When we can view life either as a celebration or a lesson, the practice of happiness becomes easier, not because there are fewer challenges, but because we *perceive* them as opportunities to help us grow.

STAGE THREE: THE REVIEW

Just as with a performance or event, it's important to take time to review how it went after a difficult situation to see what we did well and where there is room for improvement. Keep in mind however, that this is a stage of self-reflection, not self-criticism.

In this Review stage, we examine whether we were distracted when we intended to be mindful, or if we were taking things personally and reacting from the ego when our intention was not to be oversensitive or defensive. After a particularly difficult situation or conversation, this is the time when we ask ourselves where our negative charge was coming from and seek answers within ourselves.

When we review how we did, we are looking at our *progress*, not measuring our *success*. Happiness is a practice, and growing as a person is not the kind of goal where we'll one day arrive at a state of perfection—it's a journey that constantly brings new and different challenges into our lives. This means that even as we are hard at work on self-transformation, we may at times find ourselves incapable of rising to the occasion or may slip back into habits that we know don't serve us. When this happens, we don't beat ourselves up but instead use our mistakes as helpful signs of what we need to *practice more* in the future. The more we learn about ourselves and our reactions, the more we will be able to gradually elevate our habitual responses to difficult situations to a more evolved level.

It is when we understand that happiness is a practice that we can *accept* ourselves yet *continue to improve* ourselves at the same time.

When life is hard, it's not abnormal. It doesn't mean that we are failing. We just need to practice more for it to feel *less* hard. It's like playing a video game—we practice until we level up.

The last chapter of this book is about living with hope, positivity, and gratitude every single day, because even during the times when it's not easy to be happy, we are still able to practice happiness. No matter what happens, we can still be happy, always.

FOR WHEN YOU HAVE BEEN HURT:

KEEP THE DOORS TO YOUR HEART OPEN TO LET AMAZING THINGS IN

<Self-Love>

Sometimes, you meet people who are beautiful, not just in their physical appearance, but in how warm and open they are. So much of how we perceive beauty is influenced by the way someone makes us feel. When we feel uplifted in someone's presence, there's a high chance we will find the person beautiful.

One of my good friends is one such person—the more time you spend in her presence, the more beautiful you find her. She is someone who lives her life with zest and always has ever since I've known her. Many people change over time, and she has certainly grown as a person since we first became friends, but one thing that remains consistent about her is her generosity, openness, and kindness toward people, even people she's just met. She's the kind of person who can put you at ease if you're feeling awkward at a party, and she isn't shy about giving you a hug simply because she feels like it. She's always radiantly beaming like the sun.

So I was shocked to the core when one day, she quietly told me how she had once been raped.

She had gone through one of the most traumatic and horrific experiences that anyone could ever experience, but *nobody* would ever guess it from the way she embraces life.

When she described to me what she had gone through and told me how she didn't know how to help herself until years later when she started seeing a therapist regularly, I asked her, "How is it that you are still able to be so open toward people and in the way you live life?"

Her reply made me cry, for not only was it full of incredible strength, it also conveyed deep clarity and wisdom. "If I closed myself off, I'd also be blocking out all the positivity and possibilities of life—there's so much good out there, and I want those experiences. I want to let them in."

Of course, managing to do that wasn't as easy as it might sound. "It's taken so, so much work," she told me. And I could *see* how much work she'd put in to take back power over her life—to not be a victim of her circumstances despite having felt such pain. One day, I waited for her as she went for her regular therapy session, and she showed me the homework she was assigned to do—a book that she was to read and then discuss with her therapist the next time they met.

"This is such a difficult book to read," she said as she showed it to me, flipping through the pages. She didn't mean that the words were difficult to understand, but that the book discussed beliefs and concepts that she found hard to take in. Letting go of a traumatic experience takes the kind of work that requires us to constantly look at things we might find extremely uncomfortable to examine. I have such respect for my friend for having the courage to keep diving into places that give her nightmares.

The years have been such a tough journey for her, and there are still days when it's not easy to be happy, but through it all, she remains positive and optimistic for the simple reason that although she was a victim of circumstances, she was determined to not be *victimized* by them.

In order to prevent the experience from robbing her of the happiness she knows she deserves in life, she has *actively* practiced the work of letting go, understanding, and acceptance. It's not about *trying* to forgive; it's about the understanding that as long as she holds on, she won't have the kind of peace she wants in her life.

Today, she remains my most *open* friend. Many of us are kind, friendly, and cheerful, but we can also be extremely cautious about extending our openness and warmth to others. But my friend's openness to living exemplifies who she is as a person; though she's smart and savvy in the way she approaches life and certainly takes precautions in situations that might be dangerous, she doesn't live life in a state of suspicion. She doesn't reserve her warmth and openness only for the people she knows or deems worthy but extends them to everyone she meets.

Despite having gone through some extremely painful experiences, she is still one of the *happiest* people I know due to her inner work and these qualities. Because of her openness, *a multitude of blessings* have come into her life. She attracts the best job opportunities because people adore being around her. Everyone loves being her friend—to the point that every one of her male friends has a crush on her—because we are all drawn toward the sun.

And when it comes to romantic relationships, she often gets her choice of who she wants as a partner—because she has done so much work on herself that she is able to be open and vulnerable in relationships without needing to prove anything. Over the years, she has cultivated a strong sense of self-worth, and because she respects herself, people respect her. She's worked so much on acceptance and understanding that she automatically doesn't judge or blame people, nor does she blame or judge herself for her own weaknesses. All of this translates into a level of self-awareness and maturity that is highly attractive.

People who don't know her story might think that my friend is just naturally blessed or that she was born lucky. But I know, and now you do too, that it's not about luck. The amazing experiences that we have in life are only possible because we *allow* them in. For opportunities, love, and positivity to come into our lives, we have to consciously *choose* not to build walls around ourselves.

We build walls in order to protect ourselves, but we build them so that we can live with positivity and happiness instead of negativity and hurt. So if we have walls and inner defenses, it's important to ask ourselves this question: Do our walls *succeed* at providing us with joy and happiness every single day?

Or are our walls actually more successful at keeping joy and positivity *out*? Even if we have very high walls, do we *still* find ourselves experiencing hurt and pain?

Someone once asked my mom, "If you hadn't trusted your husband so fully, do you think that would have prevented him from having an affair?"

If we ask ourselves that very same question about trust in a relationship, we will likely come to the same conclusion that my mom did at the beginning of her marriage over three decades ago: If we *want* to be in a relationship with someone, yet we *don't trust* the person, then we are only making ourselves miserable because nobody can be happy living with suspicion.

"I *chose* to trust your dad," she told me, "because I cannot be with someone I cannot trust." To her, it was that simple. "I told your dad that I chose to trust him, and that, if he were to ever betray my trust, he would have to leave."

Some people would be focused on the fact that their partner was *leaving them,* but my mom focused on how *she didn't want to be with someone she couldn't trust.* From this perspective, she didn't see herself as a victim but as someone who was making decisions for her own life and happiness.

In life, we cannot avoid hurt, pain, or negativity, simply because that is very much part of a life as a human. However, that doesn't mean that we cannot *learn* from our past experiences—every painful or negative experience we go through gives us information, either about ourselves, other people, or the environment and world we live in.

To do ourselves justice, we have to use the information and learning we gain in a *positive* manner, so we can use our past experiences to help us. We use the lessons of what we've experienced to empower ourselves by being smarter and stronger, not by allowing them to make us wary, suspicious, and fearful. While we may instinctively believe the smart thing to do is to close ourselves off in order to protect ourselves, when we think about it strategically, we know that it's not very smart to hold ourselves back by building walls.

Don't allow your experiences to make you less trusting and open, because living behind high walls perpetuates our fears and insecurities and dilutes our quality of life.

Throughout this book, I've told you stories of the adversity
my mom has faced, but the stories of the *amazing* experiences
she's had would fill another book. As with my friend, my mom's
openness to life constantly rewards her—people want to go the
extra mile for her just because they like her so much. My mom is
always getting a "yes" from people who say "no" to everyone else!

It is never more urgent to nourish and care for ourselves than
when we've experienced hurt and pain; we must either seek
help or nourish ourselves with the love and respect that has not
been given to us. Nobody can *give us* what we seek—there is no
protection against our own fears. Therefore the best gift we can
ever give ourselves is to live life with an open heart, for when the
doors to our hearts are open, we can receive the abundance of
positivity and love that comes our way.

FOR WHEN YOUR HEART IS BROKEN:
TAKE YOUR HAPPINESS BACK INTO YOUR OWN HANDS

\<Self-Love\>

No matter how old or young we are, loving someone can be extremely painful when the other person does not feel the same way.

When it comes to matters of the heart, we know that it is better for us to move on and forget someone who doesn't reciprocate our feelings, but it's hard to give up when that feeling of love seems etched into one's very soul. It sounds dramatic, but love is often the one thing that can make us forget ourselves, our dignity, our self-worth, and that we were once able to be happy before this person came along.

At this juncture, there are three main things that can help us take back our lives and live each day with joy instead of misery.

The first is to understand that when we are experiencing the feeling of love for a person, it will *seem* like there is no greater love. It will seem like we will never, ever be able to find anyone else who can even come close to how amazing this person is. But the truth is that we will *always* be able to love someone else as much or more, and there will always be people in this world who are just as amazing—or even more amazing.

If we want proof, all we have to do is look at back our past relationships. Wasn't there a time where you loved an ex so much that you couldn't bear to be apart from him or her? And now, you're living separate lives and you're completely fine, and, in fact, that person hardly even crosses your mind.

The second thing to know is that when we're "not enough for that person," it is not because we're not enough *as a person*—and we have to know the difference between the two.

Many of us believe that love is when someone *needs* us, and we take an almost personal pride in being able to make someone happy. It feels good to be the person who can be enough to "make" someone happy, but it's only possible to bring joy into someone's life, we cannot *create* joy for them. We cannot *be* someone's happiness. We cannot *be* someone's light. The most we can do is to bring our own happiness and light wherever we go.

Love is not about how much someone needs us. When someone needs us, it's not really love, it's a validation for our ego. If we equate how much someone can't live without us with love, then we will feel totally destroyed and rejected when they *can* live without us.

The third thing to know is that no one can ever, ever reject us. Don't let the word "rejection" be part of your vocabulary. People come into our lives—or don't come into our lives—for a reason. When someone breaks your heart, it is merely a very good reason why the person does not belong in your life or you in theirs— sometimes we find out later why it was not meant to be and sometimes we never know. What we *do* know, however, is that we don't have to let someone else's yardstick *measure* how worthy we are of love.

The hurt and pain from a broken heart may take time to fade, but we can always make the choice to take our hearts and our happiness back into our own hands. No matter who loves us or doesn't love us, we have to learn to love and value ourselves. It is when we are okay being alone that we draw the best and most wonderful people into our lives—it's ironic that when we don't *need* love or people to make us happy that we are at our most *attractive*. This is because people can feel the joy and warmth we bring to living life. Nothing is more attractive than someone who can take responsibility for their own happiness, because that is when we are able to be strong and confident, yet vulnerable and open at the same time.

To be with an amazing person, one has to first *be* an amazing person. When it comes to love, the best thing we can do for ourselves is to shine so brightly that the *best* people are drawn to our light.

FOR WHEN YOU'RE HAVING A BAD DAY

CHOOSE HAPPINESS, BECAUSE CHOOSING MISERY IS A LOT HARDER

<Understanding>

Sometimes, we'll wake up on the wrong side of the bed. Sometimes we'll have to go to work without having had enough sleep, after an argument with our partner, or while worrying about a family member. At times like these, it's even more important for us to center ourselves before we head out for the day by asking, "How do I want my day to be?"

We usually think of special occasions in terms of something wonderful happening, where we put on our nicest attire and bring our widest, most cheerful smiles. However, when you think about it, there is no *more* special occasion than when we're feeling down—it is precisely during these moments that we need extra help to lift ourselves up, so a bad day is the perfect day to put *more effort* into actions of positivity, whether that looks like wearing something that makes us feel good, listening to music, or smiling even wider.

It's not forced positivity when we are putting in positive actions despite not feeling good. Forcing ourselves to be positive and trying to be positive both look the same on the outside, but they feel completely different on the *inside.* When we try to lift ourselves up by initiating positive actions for ourselves, we are implementing a conscious decision based on an outcome we want. Forcing positivity, on the other hand, is pretending to be happy— an internally coerced effort based on what we think society needs us to do or how we think we should be.

Sometimes, we force ourselves to put on the appearance of being happy because we don't want people to think we're all doom and gloom. But then, when we get home, we feel even worse. If you think about it, forcing ourselves to be happy requires a lot of effort, but it's effort that doesn't pay off and only serves to further drain us.

If we're already going to be making an effort, why not channel the effort into a direction that *will* pay off? The effort can go into making a conscious choice to take positive actions. This is what it means to choose happiness—on the days when we feel bad, it's not fake or a pretense when we genuinely *try* to lift ourselves up in a positive way. If we don't make efforts to lift ourselves up, who is going to help us?

When we're having a bad day, we have to decide if we are willing for our day to get worse—because that's exactly what's going to happen if we do nothing. If we start our day at level zero and put in no effort to lift ourselves up, we're not going to *stay* at level zero—we'll be in the *negative* zone by the end of the day and will feel much, much worse. This is because negativity perpetuates negativity—not just in our own minds, but in the negative energy that people reflect back at us.

It's also important that we don't blame other people for putting us in a bad mood. People can do a multitude of things we find disagreeable, but nobody can ruin our day if we don't give others so much power. Your days are yours, so why would you allow someone else to ruin them?

When we don't choose happiness, we have to be aware that the *only* other choice is the *alternative*. And the alternative is always going to be something that costs us. We will make ourselves feel worse, make work even more torturous, or continue to attract negative experiences through our own negativity.

For example, if we don't enjoy our work, it can be hard to put in the positive actions to be happy every day, but the alternative is to have a lack of happiness every day. To put effort into being happy can be hard, but the alternative is daily misery, which is *even harder*.

What is important for us to realize is that sometimes, we *think* we have *no choice* when all along we are actually *choosing the alternative*—we have accidentally chosen the *alternative to happiness* without even realizing it. When we don't choose happiness, we are choosing misery by default.

Life is too short to pretend to be happy, and life is also too short to *stay* unhappy. So, the only thing to do is to *work* on being genuinely happy. When it comes to our goals in life, we work for them. So why is happiness any different? The work lies in taking the mental action of deciding to smile, deciding to let go, deciding to be grateful, and deciding to focus on the silver lining.

We're human, and being human means that we are going to feel sad, down, and negative, and we will experience problems and pain over the course of our lives. It's never going to be easy to just not feel sad, or to just not be negative, or to just get over our problems or pain. But the focus is not on how *hard* it is, the focus is on asking ourselves, "Well, do I want this to be how my life is forever? Or do I want to choose to try my best to rise above it, overcome it, and move forward positively so I can live each day with joy?

When we ask ourselves these questions, our thoughts may bring us to the *futility* of our situation, which might be a real-world issue that we cannot change. We may feel frustrated and think thoughts like "No! I *don't want* this to be my life! This is *why* I'm unhappy, can't you see?!"

But what we *don't* see is that while we may not be able to choose our situation, we can choose *how we live in our situation* every day.

Our life situation is not our life—there is a very significant difference between the two.

Our *life situation* is what has or has not happened to us, what we have or don't have in a material sense, and the conditions of our life. There are certain life situations that we can usually determine, like where we choose to work and whom we choose to partner with, but even then, there are certain outcomes that are out of our hands. We don't get to decide who our colleagues are, and we cannot dictate whether or not a partner will be faithful. Then, there are life situations in which we have absolutely no choice, like our family of origin, the circumstances into which we were born, or whether or not someone loves us.

What is really important for us to know is that how we choose to *feel* about our lives can be *independent* of our life situation. It is without a shred of doubt true that our life situations affect our lives, but the honest truth is that how happy or unhappy we are is not dependent upon our life situation but on how we *perceive our situation.*

The joy of living doesn't come from having the best life situation. This is why people who have gone through what seem like insurmountable challenges and pain can still live their lives with happiness and joy.

When it's hard to be happy, we have to ask ourselves if having the perfect life situation will really make us happy. If that is truly the case, then how is it possible that people who have so much can be unhappy and people who have so *little* can be so happy?

So much of our capacity to practice happiness depends on how we view life. If we think that we have been bestowed life on earth so that we can *enjoy life,* then it's going to be very hard to be happy, because not every experience in our life will be enjoyable—we have to do things that are difficult, we become sick, our hearts get broken, and all manner of accidents can happen. Our life situation is never going to be absent of problems, challenges, hurtful things, and even pain.

However, if we believe that we've been given the privilege of life so we can *live each day with joy,* then even when we don't *feel* happy in our most difficult moments, we can still understand that there is yet joy to be experienced.

Even a bad day means that we *still have days,* and that is something to be truly grateful for.

This is the truest sense of happiness—the kind of acceptance of our reality where even when our circumstances are undesirable, we do not despair.

When we allow our happiness to be easily disturbed, it means that we will always be at the mercy of whatever life decides to throw at us, in a way not unlike a puppet that allows others to pull its strings—we're happy when we have a happy experience, and we're unhappy when we have an unhappy experience.

When we choose happiness, it doesn't mean that we are able to immediately be happy, because again, happiness is a practice. We will still have bad days, and that's when we can remind ourselves to choose happiness. The alternative is misery, and being miserable is *significantly harder* than taking positive actions to lift ourselves up.

A bad day is still a good day when we can take actions, no matter how small, to live with joy. Then, our good days don't happen by chance, they happen by design.

FOR WHEN YOU'RE HAVING
A DIFFICULT TIME

REMEMBER THAT LIFE DOESN'T HAPPEN TO US, IT HAPPENS FOR US

<Acceptance>

Why must this happen to me? Is there something wrong with me? Am I being punished?

Why do difficult things happen to us? It's because that's just how life happens. There's nothing wrong with us when we experience challenges and pain. Life isn't trying to punish us when it's hard; life is just being what it is.

Why is it that when our life situations are easy and free of challenges, we can accept them easily and without resistance, but when our lives aren't easy and are fraught with challenges, we cannot accept them?

Sometimes, we think that we mustn't accept a situation because we believe life shouldn't be this way for us. Our present can be so easily ruined, tarnished, and diluted, not by other people or by our circumstances, but by our projection of how life could and should be for us.

Yet, does any one of us know what our life is *supposed* to be like? How do we know that what we are experiencing right now isn't exactly what we're meant to experience? We always feel like things should be better, but how do we know that things aren't *already better*?

Perhaps what is happening in our lives, no matter how hard or how painful, isn't happening *against* us or happening *to* us—it's happening *for* us.

I remember when I was in the car with my mom one day and we missed a turn that added another thirty minutes to our journey. We were going to be late for our meeting, which was not ideal.

Then it occurred to me: How do I know that the wrong turn wasn't a right turn? If we had taken the "correct" path and stayed on the original route, maybe we would have ended up in an accident. Perhaps going down the wrong road was life's way of helping us. Perhaps it happened *for* us. Because, given a choice, I would *gladly* take being thirty minutes late over being injured in an accident.

The thing is, when something undesirable, painful, or difficult happens to us, we suffer because. either consciously or subconsciously, we think that the alternative is better. But when you think about it, there is an equal chance that the alternative could have been *much worse.* And if we somehow knew how much worse it would have been, wouldn't we suddenly be *thankful* for our current pain?

In life, we *don't know* which reality is better—our current reality or an alternate one. When we're in pain, we wish life could be kinder, but perhaps life *is being kind.* We just don't know which of those possibilities is more likely to be true.

And here's the thing—if we *don't know* what is true, then why would we want to choose to believe in the version that causes us *more suffering*?

It is not a partner or ex-lover who destroyed our lives. It is not our upbringing that is holding us back from greatness. It is our belief in how things should have happened *differently* that is causing us such stress, distress, jealousy, anger, frustration, and sadness.

Maybe if someone you love hadn't betrayed you, you wouldn't have left a relationship that would have turned out to be toxic for your health. Maybe if you hadn't encountered heartbreak or pain, you would always have depended on someone else for your happiness instead of learning to value and love yourself. Maybe if you hadn't lost that job, you would feel incredibly trapped a few years later and would have missed other opportunities when they came knocking. Maybe if you hadn't been hurt, you wouldn't understand what kindness means. Maybe if you hadn't made that mistake today, you would have made the mistake later, when it mattered even more and had even more dire consequences.

When something undesirable happens to us, it's hard to believe that anything positive might come out of it. But there is always a reason for everything, though sometimes we don't see it yet.

The truth is, we may never know for sure why we need to experience the difficulties and challenges in our lives. Yet, if we choose to believe that life happens *for* us, it means we are making a *conscious choice* to perceive challenges as something beneficial so that we can navigate through them in the most productive and positive way.

When we believe that life happens for us, it also means that we are choosing to see life as either a celebration or a lesson, so that whatever happens, we win—we are either happy and joyous or we're growing as a person. This means that when challenges come, we will not suffer due to questioning why or wishing that things were different. Instead, we will not only accept but embrace our challenges because we see them as blessings meant to help us better understand ourselves and the people around us.

Are we blessed? We may never be sure. Do we *feel blessed*? For this question, we can decide the answer.

It's almost strange how it is impossible to change external reality, yet whatever it is we choose to believe in *becomes our reality*. So when life is difficult for us, we can always choose to believe that it's happening *for* us, rather than against us, because that is the belief that brings more peace instead of more suffering. When we shift our perception of our lives, nothing changes, yet *everything* changes.

FOR WHEN YOU WANT TO BE EASILY HAPPY:

MAKE EVEN
THE SIMPLE THINGS
A FIVE-STAR EXPERIENCE

<Perspective>

"Thank you." "Thank you." "Thank you." That's what I remember my late grandmother saying the most. Every single time I saw my grandma, she would hold my hand and say, "thank you" without fail. I remember always laughing and asking her, "Why are you thanking me? I didn't do anything!"

I started to realize that my grandma wasn't thanking me for anything I did, she said "thank you" so often because she felt grateful for her family and for her life, and she wanted a way to express that.

That was why my grandma's life was always so rich. She had very little money and worked herself to the bone supporting a family of ten children, but she never once thought her life wasn't good—she felt blessed every single day until she passed away.

Out of all the lessons in my life, this is the one that I cherish the most. The lesson is that it truly doesn't matter whether we have very little or a lot—what matters is the *gratitude* we have within us for what we do have.

When you think about it, we're not actually *happier* when we have more, largely due to the fact that anything amazing very quickly becomes normal for us. We get *used* to things and even to people. There's a honeymoon phase with everything we experience, especially our relationships. The pleasure always dwindles.

This is why having more vacations, more money, and a more luxurious lifestyle doesn't make us *happier*—life is such that our level of happiness always comes back to equilibrium.

Due to this leveling effect, if we spend our lives pursuing *more*, we may find it harder and harder to feel fulfilled because the benchmark of what is required to make us happy rises higher and higher until it's more and more difficult to find new and exciting things to beat the enjoyment, excitement, and pleasure we previously had. We often subconsciously *compare* our present experiences to our past experiences, and our mind may follow the path of thinking, "It could have been better."

Ironically, when we have higher standards in life, we may sabotage our own happiness without even realizing it, because comparison is the greatest thief of joy. When we habitually measure and compare our experiences, we become harder to please, which means it is then more difficult for us to take joy in the small things. If we're harder to please, it means that we are making our happiness more conditional.

It used to be a running joke in my marriage that my husband is too easily pleased. I love gourmet ice cream, while Yuri is totally happy with simple vanilla from the grocery store. I like my coffee hot, while he still enjoys his when it has gone cold. I can cook him the same meal day after day, and, not only does not he not get bored eating it, he's *happy* to eat the same thing every single day.

It's not that Yuri has no preferences or standards—he can definitely tell that a piping hot pizza is tastier than a soggy cold pizza!—but it's that he finds *the same level of enjoyment* in both scenarios.

I noticed that Yuri was often the *happier* eater between the two of us. This was when I really thought about it: wouldn't it be such a *joy*, I mused, to be so easily pleased?

I've always taken such pride in my tastes and standards that I had to stop and re-evaluate if they were actually holding me back from being easily delighted and easily grateful. I realized then that being easily pleased is such a blessing, because it's a wonderful way to practice gratitude. Being easily pleased doesn't mean that we cannot enjoy the good things in life; it means that we can *easily find the joy* in our experiences.

Being aware of this doesn't mean that we shouldn't enjoy life—it is a blessing to have wonderful experiences—it means we can consciously decide to be someone who is easily pleased as opposed to someone who is hard to please. We don't want to let our love for fine gourmet food dilute our happiness when we eat a simple meal from a taco truck or let the experience of flying first class turn us into someone who finds it hard to be happy when flying coach.

When we are easily pleased, it means that our minds can automatically find the opportunity for gratitude in even the *smallest* things. Then, every experience is a five-star experience!

It is when we can find the *same level* of enjoyment and happiness regardless of the experience that we are truly blessed. This is why something as simple as saying "thank you" can do so much for our happiness—it's never for the person or for the thing that we say thank you, but rather it helps us to see normal things, and even old things, with *new eyes.*

And *this* sort of appreciation is priceless. Because no matter what we have or who we have, it is *gratitude* which makes people and things priceless and makes our lives richer, better, and happier.

It is a worthy goal to be someone who is easily pleased and easily delighted, someone who says "thank you" *all* the time to everyone and to all things great and small, every single day. Because then, as it was for my grandma, it is *very* possible to be happy, always.

Acknowledgements

Thank you, thank you, thank you. Thank you for reading this. Thank you to every single one of you from my *Be Happy, Always* community online and offline who have been on this journey of growth with me.

People always ask me how I became the person I am today, and now I want to thank and introduce to you the three people whose wisdom have influenced me the most.

To Sue Chan, I am so lucky that out of all the people in this world, you chose to let me into your life and your heart. Having you in my life has inspired me and taught me so much about the actions I needed to take to create change in my life. Seeing how you love your mother taught me so much about how to love mine, and for this alone I will never be able to adequately express my gratitude (though I will keep trying!). This book would not be what it is without you helping me grow. Thank you for being my best friend, my business partner, and a beautiful human being.

Sue and I collaborated to develop the Expectation Circle in chapters two and three, which is a testament to how amazing she is and how much fun we have working together.

To my husband, Yuri Wong, thank you for loving me, inspiring me, accepting me, and never giving up on me! You have taught me so much through your sheer determination to be a better person. It was Yuri's idea to turn my writing into short video clips to be shared online. Thank you, my love, for encouraging me to do what I love and for your belief in me as a person. So many of the lessons in this book are what we've practiced together. It is through our relationship that I keep learning so much about myself and about love. Your willingness to understand me is a kind of love that I don't take for granted. To be able to grow old with you is an adventure.

To my mom, Suzen Ho, I've always said that I must have done something right to be given the gift of having someone like you as my mom in this lifetime. Because you are also my best friend, I've always felt like I never needed anything or anyone to feel loved. Thank you for telling me that I can always come to you no matter what trouble I find myself in and for making me feel like you *always* have my back without judgement. Thank you for loving me enough to go through the discomfort of telling me things that you know I won't like to hear, yet are incredibly necessary for me to know. Even though my initial reactions may not always show it, your advice and guidance are more valuable than gold. Thank you for always making sure I know how worthy and how loved I am and always balancing that out with making sure I reflect and take responsibility for what I can improve on. Thank you for painstakingly reading my drafts and giving me such valuable feedback! Writing this book is important to me because it means that I get to capture your stories and spirit in print forever.

To Mark and Sarah Teng, Terimunite Lournard Chandran, and his mother, Mary Lourdes-Chandran, thank you for being so open and allowing me the privilege of sharing your stories!

To my brother, Sean Ooi, to the sister of my heart, Lim Sing Yi, and to my parents-in-law, Dad Wong Meng Kiang and Mum Irene Wong, thank you for loving me as you do. To my dearest friend Carolyn Geh, thank you for always inspiring me with your positivity. A special shout-out to Joshua Wong for your moral support and for buying me copious amount of coffee over the months of writing this book!

To my dearest friend and designer extraordinaire Cheah Wei Chun—thank you for designing this beautiful cover! You always come through for me whenever I need help and I will never take your friendship, your support and your generosity for granted. You are a treasure and always my secret (or not-so-secret!) weapon!

Lastly, thank you to Shawn and Brenda from Mango Publishing, for being so patient and supportive and for giving me such an amazing opportunity and platform to write and publish this.

About the Author

Journalist, television host, and motivational speaker Xandria Ooi grew up in Malaysia, one of the sunniest parts of the world. Her writing career started in high school and continued all through university, where she penned articles and was a columnist with Malaysia's leading English newspaper, *The Star*, for fifteen years. When it was time to decide on her career, after graduating from the University of Melbourne with a degree in Economics and Finance, Xandria ventured to take a less conventional path—she continued her writing in journalism and challenged herself to host and produce regional television programs. Her first book, *Love, Work, and Everything in Between*, was published by MPH Publications in 2009.

Expanding her skills to radio, Xandria produced and hosted the breakfast show for Malaysia's first women's station, CapitalFM. Her show carried interviews and stories that served as a platform for empowering women.

In 2016, Xandria started writing short inspirational pieces about happiness and turning them into videos. She started releasing her videos each day on YouTube and Facebook and amassed fans from all over the world who resonated with her approach to living life with happiness, earning her the title of *Happiness Guru*. Fans have referred to her as "the Asian Oprah."

Xandria has a thirty-day happiness program which is available online, and she travels regularly for speaking engagements, trainings, and workshops. For regular doses of happiness, follow Xandria on Instagram (@xandriaooi), where she shares bite-sized perspectives and reminders. Xandria is married to musician Yuri Wong, and the couple candidly share their relationship ups and downs with close to a million followers in their weekly *live* video chats on Facebook (www.facebook.com/xandriaooi).

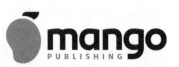

Mango Publishing, established in 2014, publishes an eclectic list of books by diverse authors—both new and established voices— on topics ranging from business, personal growth, women's empowerment, LGBTQ studies, health, and spirituality to history, popular culture, time management, decluttering, lifestyle, mental wellness, aging, and sustainable living. We were recently named 2019's #1 fastest growing independent publisher by Publishers Weekly. Our success is driven by our main goal, which is to publish high quality books that will entertain readers as well as make a positive difference in their lives.

Our readers are our most important resource; we value your input, suggestions, and ideas. We'd love to hear from you—after all, we are publishing books for you!

Please stay in touch with us and follow us at:

Facebook: Mango Publishing

Twitter: @MangoPublishing

Instagram: @MangoPublishing

LinkedIn: Mango Publishing

Pinterest: Mango Publishing

Sign up for our newsletter at www.mango.bz and receive a free book!

Join us on Mango's journey to reinvent publishing, one book at a time.